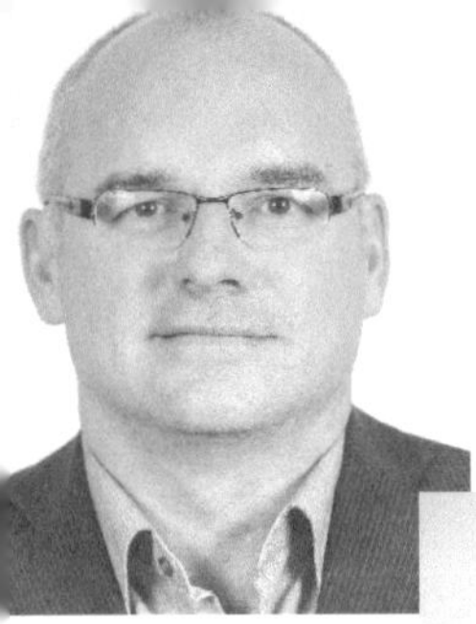
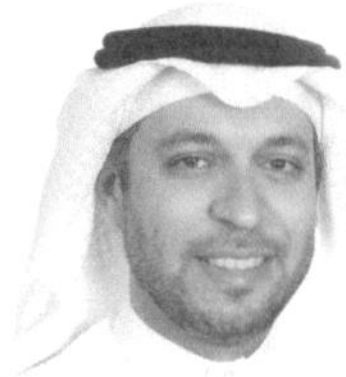
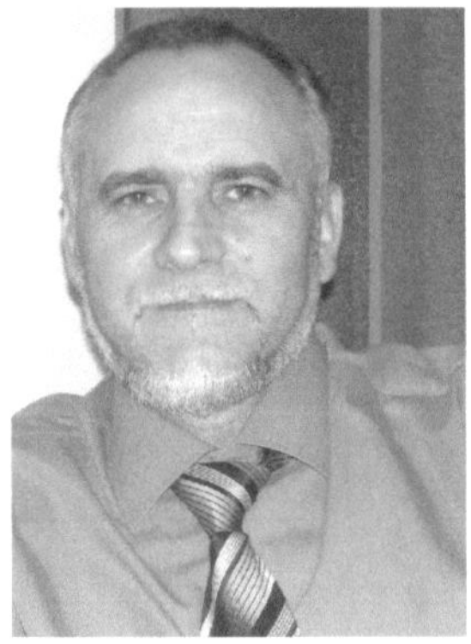
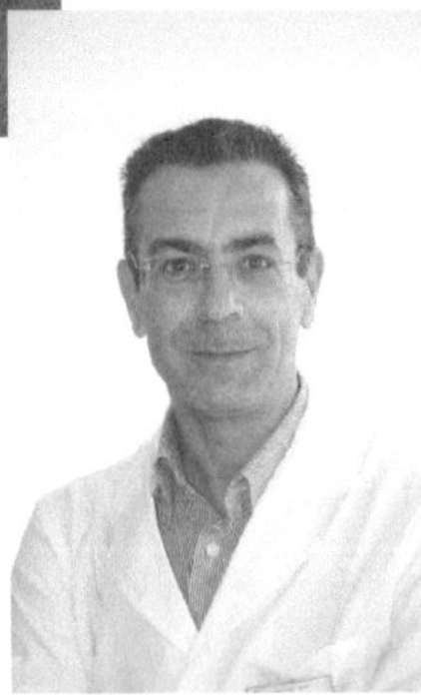
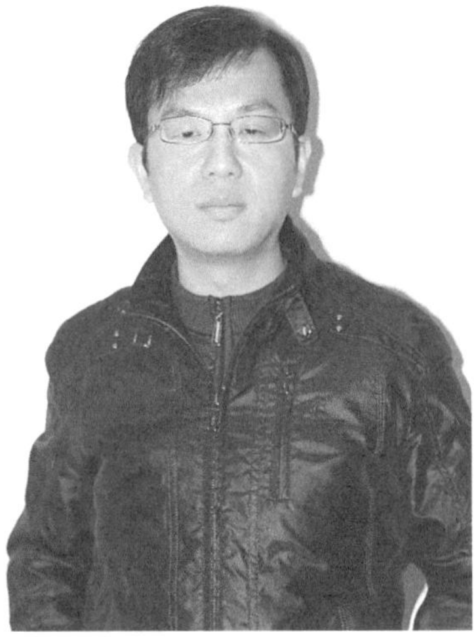
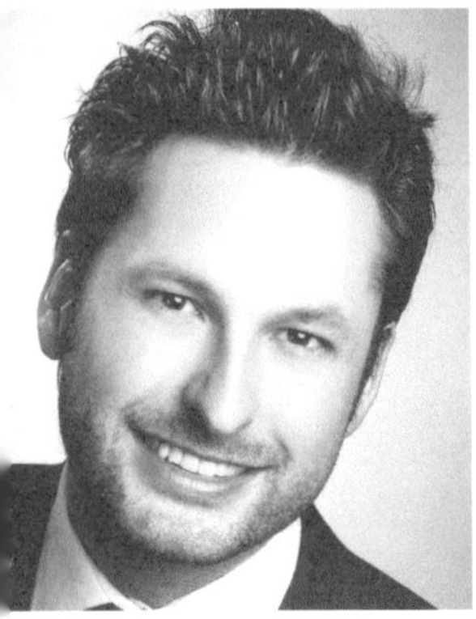
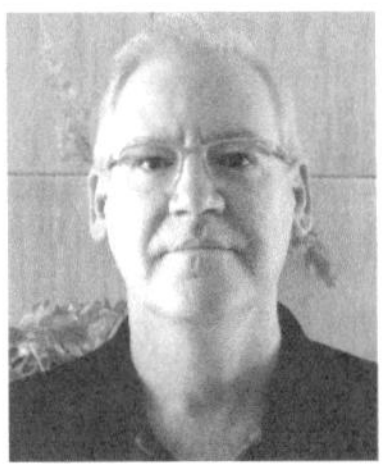

IntechOpen

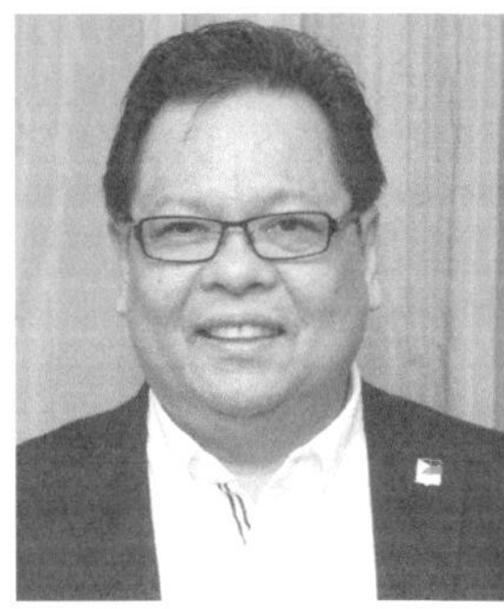
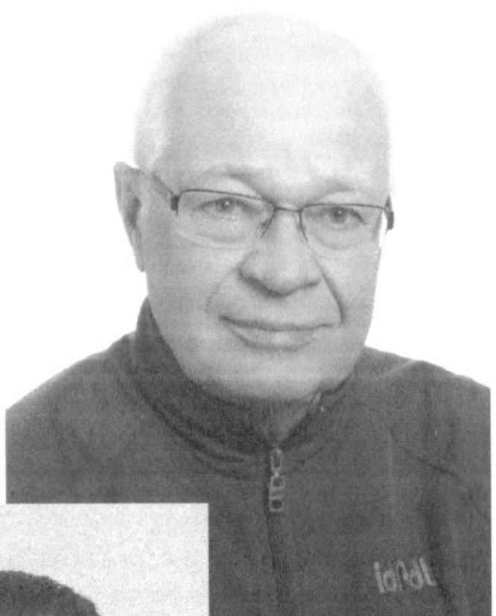
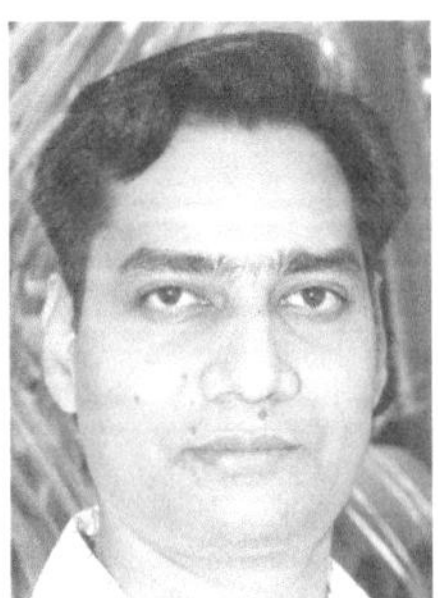
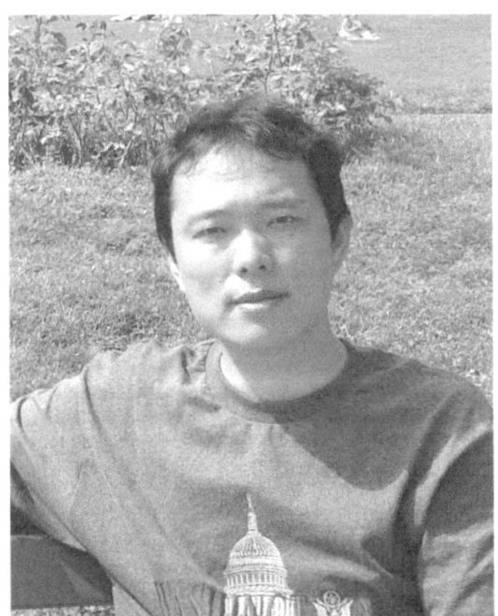
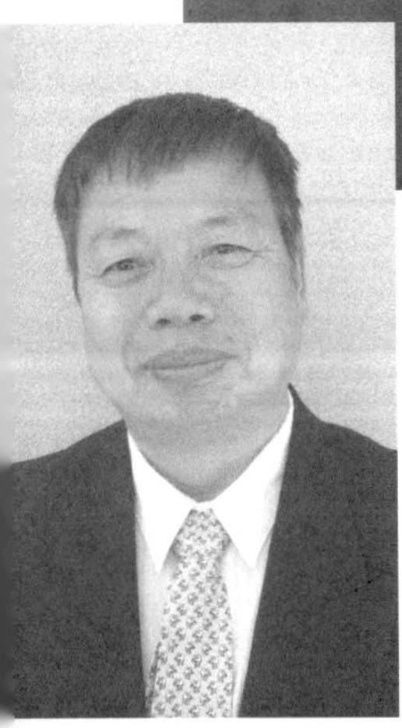
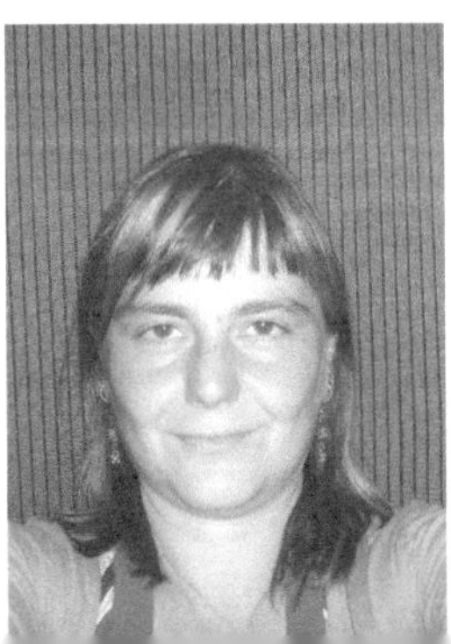

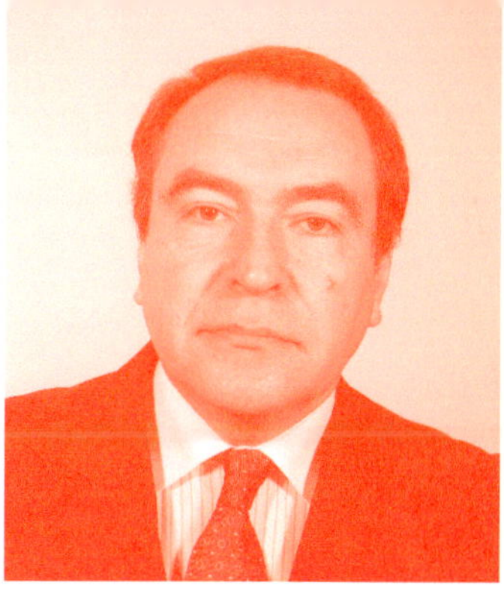
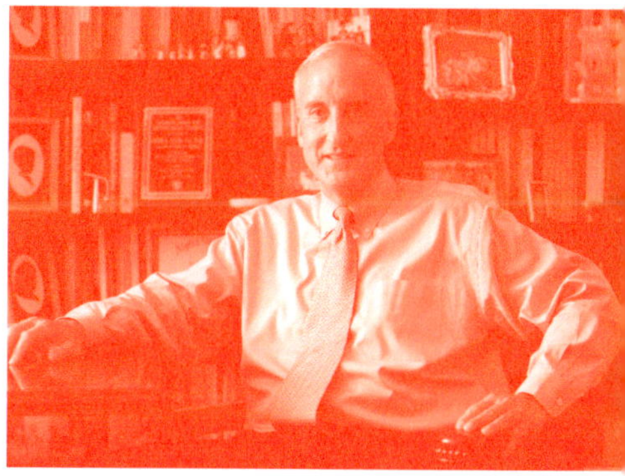
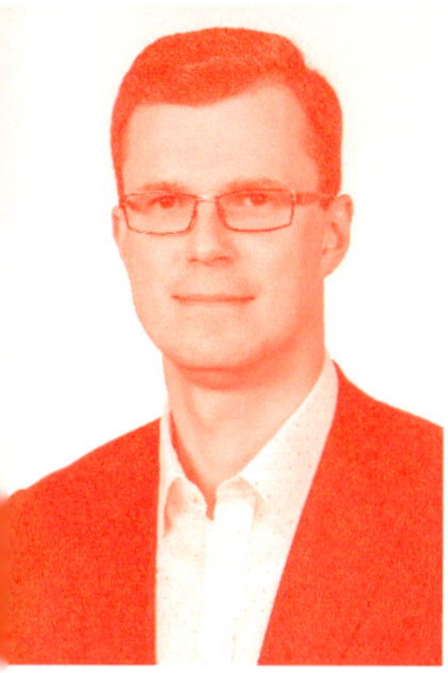
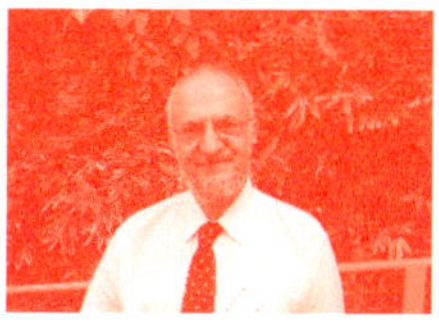
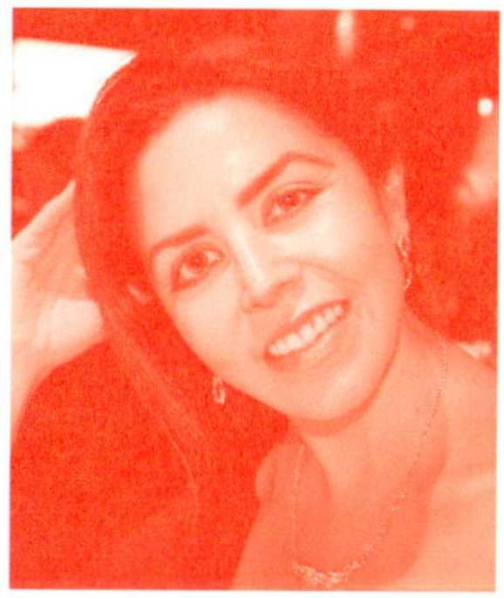

Supporting open minds since 2005

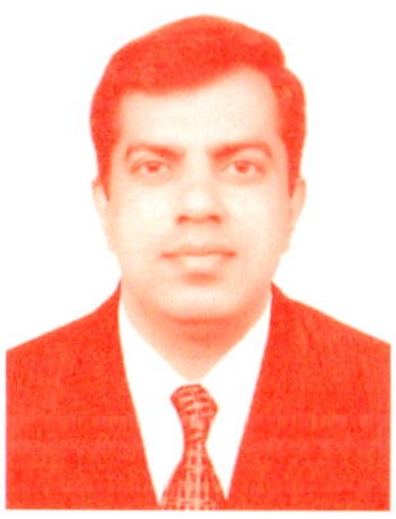
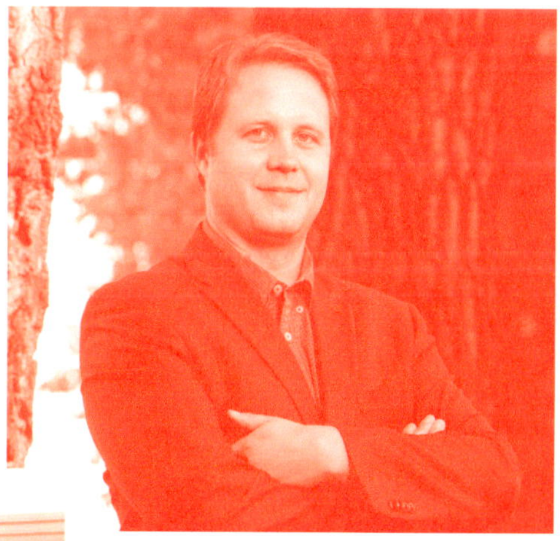
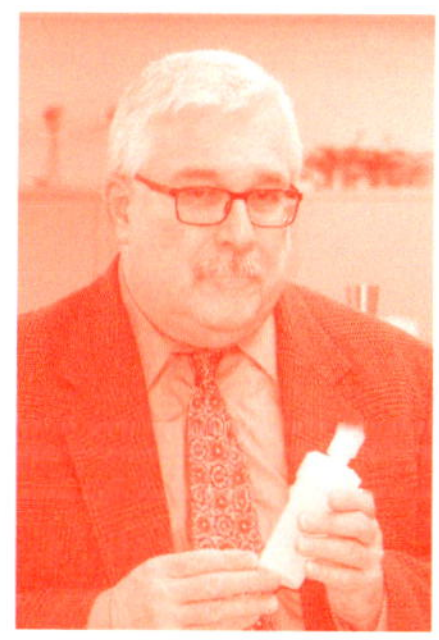
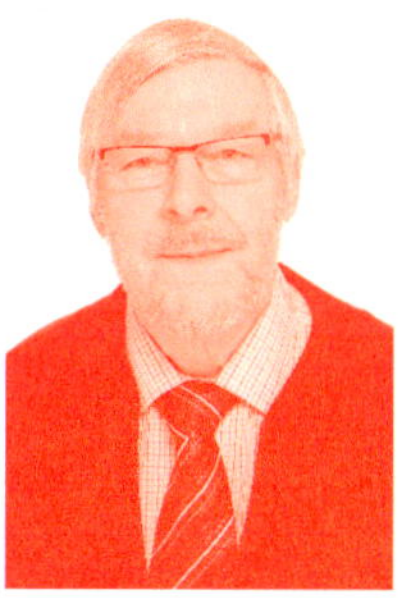
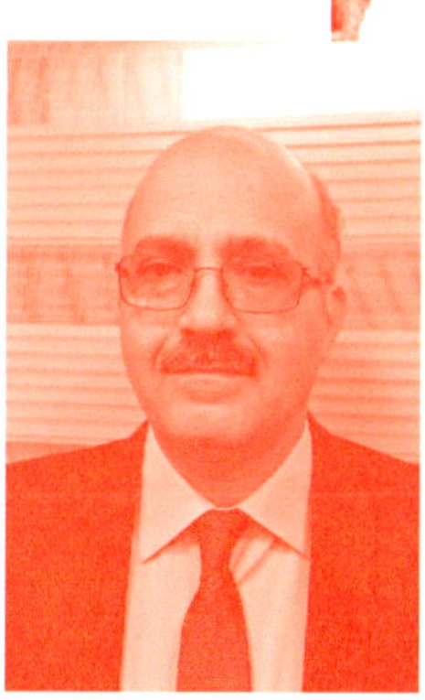
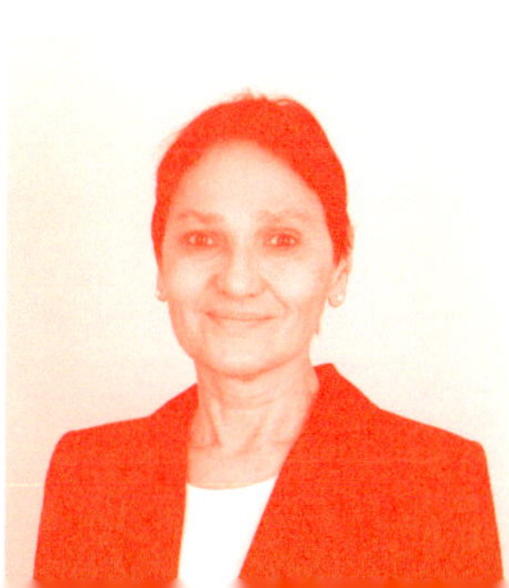
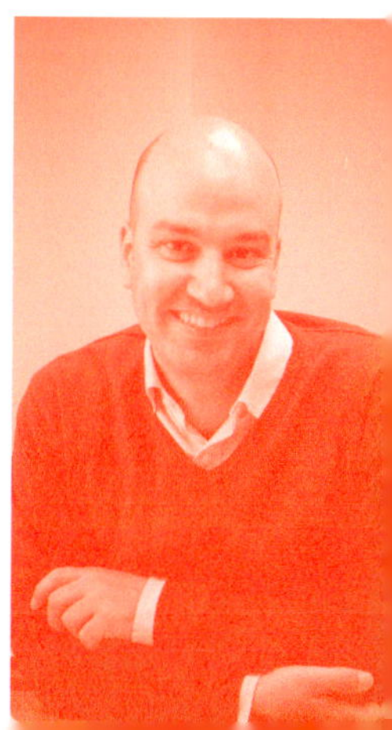

Hot Topics in Endocrinology and Metabolism
http://dx.doi.org/10.5772/intechopen.90963
Edited by Hassan Massoud Heshmati

Contributors
Valentine Suteau, Patrice Rodien, Mathilde Munier, Priya Gupta, Archisman Mahapatra, Anjali Suman, Rahul Kumar Singh, Rafael Moreno-Gómez-Toledano, María I. Arenas, Sandra Sánchez-Esteban, Alberto Cook, Marta Saura, Ricardo J. Bosch, Hassan M. Heshmati, Sara Al-Ghadban, Mary L. Teeler, Bruce A. Bunnell

First published in London, United Kingdom, 2021 by IntechOpen
IntechOpen is the global imprint of INTECHOPEN LIMITED, registered in England and Wales, registration number: 11086078, 5 Princes Gate Court, London, SW7 2QJ, United Kingdom
Printed in Croatia

British Library Cataloguing-in-Publication Data
A catalogue record for this book is available from the British Library

Additional hard and PDF copies can be obtained from orders@intechopen.com

Hot Topics in Endocrinology and Metabolism
Edited by Hassan Massoud Heshmati
p. cm.
Print ISBN 978-1-83962-911-2
Online ISBN 978-1-83962-912-9
eBook (PDF) ISBN 978-1-83962-913-6

Meet the editor

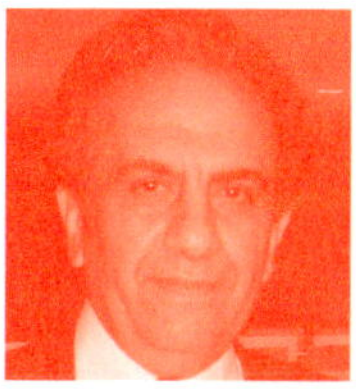

Dr. Hassan Massoud Heshmati is an endocrinologist with 45 years of experience in clinical research in academia (university-affiliated hospitals in Paris, France, and the Mayo Foundation, Rochester, MN, USA) and pharmaceutical companies (Sanofi, Malvern, PA; Essentialis, Carlsbad, CA; and Gelesis, Boston, MA, USA). His research focuses on pituitary tumors, hyperthyroidism, thyroid cancers, osteoporosis, diabetes, and obesity. He has extensive knowledge in the development of anti-obesity products. Dr. Heshmati is the author of 288 abstracts, chapters, and articles related to endocrinology and metabolism. He is currently a consultant at Endocrinology Metabolism Consulting, LLC, Anthem, AZ, USA.

Contents

Preface

Endocrine-disrupting chemicals (EDCs) represent a heterogeneous group of exogenous chemicals that interfere with the action of hormones. Their number has markedly increased over the past 60 years. EDCs may be significant components of the environmental origin of several medical conditions. The coronavirus disease 2019 (COVID-19) pandemic has affected human health around the world. Several endocrine and metabolic systems can be impacted by COVID-19. This book examines the impacts of EDCs and the COVID-19 pandemic on human health, including endocrine and metabolic consequences.

The book contains six chapters by authors from France, India, Spain, and the United States. I would like to thank all of them. I would also like to thank the great assistance of Ms. Romina Rovan at IntechOpen who supervised this book project.

Hassan Massoud Heshmati, MD
Endocrinology Metabolism Consulting, LLC
Anthem, AZ, USA

Section 1

Endocrine-Disrupting Chemicals

Chapter 1

G-Protein Coupled Hormone Receptors of the Hypothalamic-Pituitary-Gonadal Axis are Targets of Endocrine Disrupting Chemicals

Valentine Suteau, Patrice Rodien and Mathilde Munier

Abstract

Endocrine-disrupting chemicals have received significant concern, since they ubiquitously persist in the environment and are able to induce adverse effects on health, and more particularly on reproductive function. Most of the studies focused on nuclear hormone receptors as mediators of sex steroid hormones signaling. However, there are increasing evidences that peptides hormones of the Hypothalamo-Pituitary-Gonadal axis are targets of endocrine-disrupting chemicals (as Gonadotropin-Releasing Hormone, Follicle-Stimulating Hormone, Luteinizing Hormone…). The majority of these hormones act on G protein-coupled membrane receptors. This review summarizes the effects of endocrine-disrupting chemicals on homeostasis of peptides hormone of Hypothalamo-Pituitary-Gonadal axis and on their G protein-coupled membrane receptors signaling revealed by experimental, clinical, and epidemiological studies in human.

Keywords: G-protein coupled hormone receptors, hypothalamic-pituitary-gonadal axis, hormones, endocrine-disrupting chemicals

1. Introduction

Public concern of endocrine-disrupting chemicals (EDCs) has been rising since the 1990s. EDCs are defined as "an exogenous substance or mixture that alters function(s) of the endocrine system and consequently causes adverse health effects in an intact organism, or its progeny, or (sub)populations" [1–3]. EDCs are found in many products comprising plasticizers, personal care products, pesticides… [1]. Humans are constantly exposed to several different EDCs by ingestion, inhalation, and dermal contact. Some classes of EDCs have been studied in detail. Here, we selected three classes of EDCs based on knowledge of their effects on Hypothalamo-Pituitary-Gonadal (HPG) axis: bisphenol A (BPA), phthalates and dichlorodiphenyltrichloroethane (DDT). BPA is one of the most massively produced EDC with over three million tons manufactured annually [4]. It is used in food packaging, toys, resins used in canned, and medical equipment. Because its incomplete polymerization and its release from polycarbonate at high temperature, exposure to BPA is important *via* food containers [5–7]. Phthalates are used as liquid plasticizers found in a wide range of products including plastics, coatings, toys, cosmetics, and medical tubing. They are classified in two groups: high molecular weight phthalates, such as diethylhexyl phthalte (DEHP), and low molecular weight phthalates, such as dibutyl phthalates (DBP) [8]. DDT, an organochlorine pesticide, was largely used after the Second World War for its insecticidal properties. Although it was banned in the 1970s in the Western World, it continues to be used in developing countries. DDT is a synthetic mixture of three isoforms: p,p'DDT, o,p'DDT and p,p'DDD. EDCs are originally thought to act through nuclear hormone receptors, such as estrogen receptor (ER) or androgen receptor (AR) [9]. During the last decade, we, and others, were interested in the effect of EDCs on G-protein-coupled hormone receptors (GPCRs). These studies have shown that there are chemical compounds in the environment capable of binding to GPCRs and disrupting the activity and intracellular signaling pathways of receptor. Moreover, EDCs may alter pathways involved in hormone biosynthesis and/or receptor signaling regulation. This review summarizes the effects of three classes of EDCs on hormones homeostasis and GPCRs signaling involved in the HPG axis. Several molecular mechanisms can be involved in the EDC effects on the HPG axis. All studies cited here were performed in human species.

2. GPCRs implicated in the HPG axis

The GPCRs are the largest family of cell-surface receptors with over 800 members accounting for 4% of the encoded human genome [10]. About half of them have sensory functions, mediating olfaction, taste, light perception, and pheromone signaling. The other half (~350–400) are called endo-receptors, i.e. receptors that interact with endogenous ligands [11]. These receptors are involved in the detection of many extracellular stimuli (from photons or ions to large hormones proteins). Thus, they have important roles in various physiological systems. Dysfunction of GPCRs contributes to many human diseases and GPCRs represent 34% of all Food and Drug Administration-approved drugs [12].

GPCRs are characterized by a common structure with seven transmembrane helices with an extracellular N terminus and an intracellular C terminus [13]. The N-terminal portion, or transmembrane domain, constitute the ligand binding site while the C-terminal portion and the intracellular loops form a coupling domain with the intracellular effectors [14].

In the classical GPCR signaling pathway, after ligand binding, activated-GPCR binds the intracellular heterotrimeric G proteins, promoting the release of GDP from the Gα subunit, exchanged for GTP and the dissociation of the GTP-bound α subunit from βγ dimers. The activated G proteins can then transduce and amplify GPCR signals via second messengers to produce a variety of cell responses [15]. Briefly, G*αs* activates adenylyl cyclases to catalyze the conversion of ATP to cAMP. Members of the Gαi family primarily inhibit cAMP production. The $G\alpha_{q/11}$ family converts phosphatidylinositol 4,5-bisphosphate to diacylglycerol and inositol 1,4,5-trisphosphate to activate Protein Kinase C and increases intracellular Ca^{2+} levels. Approximately 10% of GPCRs can be coupled with different types of Gs subunit depending on cell type and context [16]. The second messengers then target other enzymes such as cAMP-dependent protein kinase A (PKA), GMP-dependent protein kinase G (PKG), Ca^{2+}-dependent protein kinase C (PKC) or calcium-sensitive enzymes. The Gβγ subunit can also activate a multitude of effectors (GRKs, ion channels, PI3K, phospholipases, MAP kinases) to induce a variety of cellular effects [17]. G protein-mediated signaling is discontinued when the Gα subunit hydrolyzes GTP to GDP, due to its intrinsic GTPase activity. This then leads to the reassociation of Gα with Gβγ to form the inactive heterotrimer [14]. In addition to canonical signaling through heterotrimeric G proteins, some of GPCRs can use alternative modes of GPCR activation and initiate G protein–independent pathway. The main independent pathway involves a coupling with β-arrestin. Originally, β-arrestin was identified as an essential factor in the endocytosis and arrest of GPCR signaling induced by heterotrimeric G proteins. Today, other functions associated with β-arrestins are being studied and coupling to β-arrestins is increasingly described as "scaffolding" proteins involved in multiple G protein-independent signaling pathways. Indeed, in addition to clathrin, β-arrestins are able to bind to many proteins involved in different signaling pathways (Src, ERK1/2 and JNK3 kinases protein phosphatases, ubiquitin ligases...) [18]. The activation of β-arrestins signaling pathways can take place at the membrane but also in intracellular after internalization [15]. Indeed, a growing amount of evidence suggests that several molecules have not been known to be regulated by G proteins, suggesting that β-arrestin-mediated signaling pathways may be functioning in parallel with G-protein-mediated pathways enhancing GPCR signaling pathways.

The Hypothalamo-Pituitary-Gonadal axis is active in the midgestational fetus and after birth at the minipuberty but is mainly reactivate at onset of puberty. Some receptors of the HPG axis belong to the subfamily of GPCR: gonadotropin-releasing hormone receptor (GnRHR), GPR54/Kisspeptin receptor, Neurokinin B receptor (NK3R), Prokineticin receptor (PROKR2), follicle stimulating hormone receptor (FSHR), human chorionic gonadotropin/luteinizing hormone receptor (hCG/LHR) and Relaxin Family Peptide Receptor 2 (RXFP2).

The GnRH, a neuropeptidic hormone, is secreted by hypothalamic GnRH-expressing neurons into the portal blood vessels in rhythmic pulses [19]. It binds to a membrane receptor, the GnRH receptor, also known as the luteinizing hormone releasing hormone receptor (LHRHR), on pituitary gonadotropic cells and stimulates the biosynthesis and secretion of LH and FSH [19]. GnRHR is predominantly coupled to the Gq-protein [20]. GnRH/GnRHR pathway constitutes the initial step in the HPG axis and controls reproduction in both sexes. GnRH loss-of-function mutations are associated to normosmic hypogonadotropic hypogonadism [21]. GnRH neurons appear to be directly regulated by Kisspeptin-1 (KISS1), with Neurokinin B (NKB) and Prokineticin 2 (PROK2). KISS1 is a peptidic hormone mostly expressed in the hypothalamus [22]. It activates GPR54/KISS1R, which results in the activation of phospholipase C *via* Gq [12]. GPR54 has been described in brain regions, including hypothalamus, but also in peripheral regions [22]. Kisspeptin/GPR54 pathway has a crucial role in the onset of puberty, the regulation of sex hormone mediated secretion of FSH/LH, and in the control of fertility [22, 23]. Inactivating and activating mutations in *KISS1* or *GPR54* genes have been associated with hypogonadotropic hypogonadism and precocious puberty, respectively [23].

Gonadal function is under pituitary control *via* the gonadotropin hormones: follicle stimulating hormone (FSH) and luteinizing hormone (LH) [24]. FSH and LH are synthesized and secreted by the pituitary gonadotropic cells and work together in the reproductive system. The human chorionic gonadotropin (hCG) is secreted by the placenta and controls ovarian function during gestation. LH and hCG share the same GPCR, the hCG/LHR. The FSH and hCG/LH receptor belong to the glycoprotein-hormone receptor family. Activation of the LH and FSH receptor results in the production of intracellular cyclic AMP (cAMP) *via* $G\alpha_s$ proteins [25, 26]. However, FSHR and LHR can also couple to several other effectors such as $G\alpha_q$ and β-arrestin [26–28]. FSHR is expressed in Sertoli and granulosa cells in male and female gonads, respectively, and is required for normal spermatogenesis and growth and maturation of ovarian follicles, as well as for estrogen production [29]. In women, LHR induces luteinization of granulosa cells, progesterone synthesis and *corpus luteum* maintenance during the luteal phase [30]. In men, LH stimulates testosterone production by Leydig cells [30].

Steroid hormones (estrogen, progesterone, and testosterone) secreted by the gonads, bind, and activate nuclear receptors. However, a membrane associated estrogen receptor (GPER) has been identified 15 years ago [31, 32]. Activation of GPER induces intracellular calcium mobilization, cAMP production and phosphorylation cascade involving $ERK_{1/2}$, PKA, PI3K [33]. This receptor is implicated in many physiological functions: uterine proliferation, metabolism, cardiovascular, immune, and neural system.

More recently, the INSL3/RXFP2 system pathway was identified for its role in reproduction. Insulin-like peptide-3 (INSL3) belongs to the insulin/relaxin family of peptidic hormones [34, 35]. This hormone is mainly produced by testicular Leydig cells and the production is dependent on the state of Leydig cell differentiation [34]. INSL3 is considered as a marker for Leydig cells function. Its best characterized role is in the control of testicular descent since *INSL3* gene inactivation males have bilateral cryptorchidism with testis remaining in abdominal position [36, 37].

3. Effects of EDCs on signaling of HPG axis G-protein coupled receptors

Effects of EDCs on the activity of HPG axis GPCR identified in the literature search are summarized in **Table 1**.

3.1 Hypothalamic hormones receptor

Currently, there are no data on the effects of EDCs on the activity of human hypothalamic hormone receptors. However, some studies have been conducted with animal models. Exposure to phthalates leads to a modulation of GnRHR expression (positive or negative depending on the studies) [50, 51], as well as an increase in its expression in rat uterus [52].

3.2 Gonadotropin hormones receptor

EDCs, like phthalates, increase the FSHR expression in human granulosa cells [38]. DDT has been shown to disturb the FSH induced-cAMP accumulation [39] and aromatase activity in human granulosa cells [40]. Recently, we showed that DDT behaves as an FSHR positive allosteric modulator [41]. DDT interacts with the receptor in the minor binding pocket in the transmembrane domain. DDT acts on the early steps of activation of the FSHR and induces an increase in FSH-stimulated cAMP production. Moreover, the binding of DDT enhances the FSHR response to hCG. The increased response to FSH in the presence of DDT and the gain of sensitivity to hCG may therefore by deleterious. In opposite, BPA is a FSHR negative allosteric modulator [41].

As for FSHR, EDCs, like BPA, disturbes the expression of hCG/LHR in human endometrial stromal cells [42]. In CHO-K1 cells stably transfected with hCG/LHR, DDT reduced the cAMP accumulation induced by hCG [39, 41] and hLH (Munier et al., Arch Toxicol, in revision). Moreover, DDT decreases the hCG- and hLH-promoted β-arrestin 2 recruitment (Munier et al., Arch Toxicol, in revision). DDT seems to act as a negative allosteric modulator of the hCG/LHR signaling.

GPCR	EDC	Study model	Main results	
FSHR	DBP [10^{-7} *to* 10^{-4} *M*]	Human granulosa cells	DBP increases FSHR expression	[38]
	DDT [10^{-7} *to* 10^{-4} *M*]	CHO-K1 - hFSHR	DDT decreases cAMP production stimulated by FSH	[39]
	DDE [10^{-7} *to* 10^{-4} *M*]	Human granulosa cells from IVF	DDE potentiates the FSH induced aromatase activity	[40]
	DDT [10^{-7} *to* 10^{-5} *M*]	CHO-K1 - hFSHR	DDT is an FSHR positive allosteric modulator	[41]
	BPA [10^{-5} *M*]	CHO-K1 - hFSHR	BPA decreases cAMP production stimulated by FSH	[41]
hCG/ LHR	BPA [10^{-6} *M*]	Human endometrial stromal cells	BPA decreases hCG/LHR expression	[42]
	DDT [10^{-7} *to* 10^{-5} *M*]	CHO-K1 - hCG/ LHR	DDT decreases cAMP production stimulated by hCG/LHR	[41]
RXFP2	DEHP [10^{-9} *to* 10^{-5} *M*]	HEK293 - hRXFP2	DEHP increases cAMP production stimulated by INSL3	[43]
	DBP [10^{-9} *to* 10^{-5} *M*]		DBP increases cAMP production stimulated by INSL3	
	BPA [10^{-11} *to* 10^{-7} *M*]	HEK293 - hRXFP2	BPA increased cAMP production stimulated by INSL3	
	DEHP + DBP + BPA [10^{-10} *to* 10^{-6} *M*]	HEK293 - hRXFP2	DEHP+DBP + BPA mixture decreases cAMP production stimulated by INSL3	
GPER	BPA [10^{-6} *M*]	Human breast cancer cells	BPA increases GPER expression	[44]
	BPA [10^{-12} *to* 10^{-9} *M*]	Human testicular seminoma cells	BPA promotes cellular proliferation *via* GPER activation	[45]
	BPA [10^{-9} *to* 10^{-5} *M*]	HEK293 - hGPER	BPA is a GPER agonist and induces the Gs protein pathway	[46]
	BPA [10^{-9} *to* 10^{-5} *M*]	Human breast and lung cancer cells; cancer-associated fibroblasts	BPA induces $ERK_{1/2}$ activation and gene expression through GPER leading to cellular proliferation and migration	[47, 48]
	BPA [10^{-7} *to* 10^{-4} *M*]	Human granulosa cells	BPA induces apoptosis *via* GPER activation	[49]
	o,p'-DDE [10^{-7} *to* 10^{-6} *M*]	Human breast cancer cells	o,p'-DDE is a GPER agonist and induces the Gs protein pathway	[32, 46]

Table 1.
Experimental studies studying the effect of EDC on HPG axis GPCR signaling.

3.3 Insl3 receptor, RXFP2

Only one study has very recently focused on the effect if EDCs on receptor signaling to INSL3: RXFP2. In a cellular model of HEK293 transiently expressing human RXFP2, individually, BPA, DEHP and DBP potentiate the cAMP response to INSL3 [43]. Because of their ubiquity, BPA, DEHP and DBP are present in many human biological fluids, as the amniotic liquid. Furthermore, everyone is chronically exposed to mixtures of environmental chemical factors resulting in toxicological interactions that cannot be predicted by reprotoxicological studies of single molecules. The combination of these three molecules, at concentrations found in human amniotic fluid, decreases the basal activity of RXFP2 as well as the response to INSL3. The structural similarity between FSHR and RXFP2 suggests that small hydrophobic molecules, like phthalates and BPA, could use the same binding sites as DDT in FSHR. The binding of one or two compounds to this site could lead to a stabilization of the active state of the receptor driving an increase of agonist activity [53]. In contrast, the binding of three compounds (DEHP+DBP + BPA) likely leads to a steric hindrance that may prevent the conformational changes necessary for the activation of RXFP2 and probably stabilize an inactive state. This study shows that in addition to individual EDC targets, HPG axis GPCRs can also be targeted by EDC cocktails.

3.4 Membrane sexual steroid hormones receptor

The G protein-coupled receptor (GPER/GPR30) is a membrane estrogen receptor [31]. Gene inactivation of *GPER* in mice did not induce major modifications in reproductive function [54]. However, several studies show that this receptor has pro-oncogenic effects in hormone-dependent cancers. Although many EDCs exhibit low binding affinities to the nuclear ERs and often require relatively high concentrations (>1 μM) to affect genomic pathways, several studies have focused on non-genomic signaling mediated by GPER [55].

Various DDT derivatives and BPA bind to GPER with a K_d between 1 to 10 μM and are competitors of E2 [46]. The binding affinity of EDCs for GPER is higher than for the nuclear receptors. Nevertheless, low concentrations of o,p'DDE and BPA increased cAMP production by GPER [32, 45, 46]. BPA and phthalate (MEHP) also affect proliferation and migration in human cervical cancer cells [56], in human seminoma cells [45], human breast cancer cells and cancer-associated fibroblasts that lack nuclear ERs [47, 57] as well as the migration and invasion of lung cancer cells [48]. BPA modifies these cellular responses by modulating different intracellular signaling pathways ($ERK_{1/2}$ or Akt phosphorylation, gene expression) through GPER activation. In opposite, GPER mediates BPA-induced intracellular stress generation (ROS production and calcium accumulation) and apoptosis (caspase activation and mitochondrial membrane potential decrease) in human granulosa cells [49]. Recently, it has also been shown that BPA increases GPER gene expression in breast cancer cell lines [44]. Finally, bisphenols AF and B, two substitutes of BPA, exert high estrogenic effects via GPER pathway at nanomolar concentrations [58, 59].

4. Effects of EDCs on the synthesis and secretion of HPG axis hormones

Effects of EDCs on the synthesis and secretion of HPG axis hormones identified in the literature search are summarized in **Table 2**.

Study population	EDC exposure	Matrix/ biomarker	Main results	
192 mother–child pairs from e-waste recycling town and 70 from control area	Free BPA in cord blood serum	*Kiss* gene expression in placenta	Higher BPA concentrations showed positive correlation with *Kiss* gene expression	[60]
73 girls with central precocious puberty and 31 controls	Seven urinary phthalate metabolites concentrations	Serum kisspeptin	Positive correlation between kisspeptin- and mono-n-butyl phthalate	[61]
535 men (18–40 yr) living or not in pesticides contamined area.	Lipid-adjusted DDE and DDT concentrations	Serum FSH, LH, T, E2	Positive association between DDT or DDE with T	[62]
749 Swedish (fishermen and their pregnant wife)	p,p′-DDE serum level	Serum FSH, LH, T, E2	Positive association between DDE and FSH or LH	[63]
97 adult men living in nothern Thailand	plasma levels of DDT and its metabolites	Serum FSH, LH, T, E2	Negative association of E2 level with p,p'-DDE and positive association with o,p'-DDE	[64]
107 males exposed to DDT in Italy	Lipid-adjusted p,p'-DDE and p,p'-DDT serum concentration	Serum FSH, LH, T, E2	No association with serum hormone levels	[65]
604 adults (men and women) in Brazil areas exposed to pesticides	Serum concentrations of 19 pesticides including p,p'-DDT and o,p'-DDT	Serum FSH, LH, T, E2	In men, o,p'-DDT level was associated with lower T, in peri- and postmenopausal women, p,p'-DDT showed inverse associations with LH; No association in premenopausal women	[66]
234 mothers and their sons	Serum o,p'- and p,p'-DDT, p,p'-DDE from mothers during pregnancy or at delivery and their sons at 9 years.	Serum FSH, LH and T in sons at 12 years	Prenatal maternal DDT and DDE levels were associated with decreases in LH	[67]
45 girls with early breast development, 16 girls with early puberty, and 33 girls with no signs of puberty	2,4-DDT and 4,4'-DDE in the serum and adipose tissue samples.	Serum basal and stimulated LH and FSH level	Basal and stimulated LH were higher in girls with detectable serum DDE levels	[68]
308 young men	Urinary BPA concentrations	Serum LH, T, E2	Higher urinary BPA concentrations were associated with increased serum T, E2, and LH	[69]
215 healthy young men (18–23 yr)	Urinary BPA concentrations	Serum FSH, LH, T, E2	Positive association between urinary BPA and LH levels	[70]

Study population	EDC exposure	Matrix/ biomarker	Main results	
560 men aged 18–55 years	Urinary BPA concentrations	Serum FSH, LH, T	BPA was associated with increased serum levels of LH and FSH in male smokers, and with decreased serum levels of total T in men with BMI ≥ 25 kg/m2.	[71]
167 men from an infertility clinic	Urinary BPA concentrations	Serum FSH, LH, T, E2	Positive association between urinary BPA and serum FSH	[72]
244 mothers-child pairs	Serum maternal total BPA concentration during second or third trimester	Serum FSH, LH, T, E2	No association with serum hormone levels	[73]
159 women with premature ovarian insufficiency and 186 controls	Urinary concentrations of BPA	Serum FSH, LH	No association with serum hormone levels	[74]
106 BPA-exposed factories and 250 unexposed female workers	Urinary concentrations of BPA	Serum FSH, LH, E2	Inverse association between BPA and FSH in unexposed group	[75]
143 healthy, premenopausal women	Urinary concentrations of BPA	Serum FSH, LH, E2	No association with serum hormone levels	[76]
172 peripubertal boys	Urinary concentrations of BPA	Serum FSH, LH, T	No association with serum hormone levels	[77]
130 children with Attention-Deficit/ Hyperactivity Disorder and 68 controls (boys and girls)	Urine levels of phthalates and BPA	Serum FSH, LH, T, E2	Among boys with ADHD, MBzP and MEHP levels were positively correlated with T; among girls, MEP was positively correlated with LH and T	[78]
136 girls (6–9 yr) with early puberty and 136 controls	Urinary BPA concentrations	Serum basal and stimulated LH and FSH level, E2	In early puberty group, negative correlation between BPA and peak FSH levels	[79]
479 pregnant women and their infants (boys and girls)	Urinary 12 phthalate metabolites concentrations at gestational week 28	Serum T, LH, FSH during mini puberty	No association with serum hormone levels	[80]
302 Korean children and adolescents	Urinary and serum concentrations of DEHP, MEHP, DBP, MBP	Serum FSH, LH, T, E2	Positive correlations between serum DBP or MEHP, and E2 and/or LH in children.	[81]

Study population	EDC exposure	Matrix/ biomarker	Main results	
106 males and females (11–88 yr)	Urinary phthalate metabolites	Serum FSH, LH, T, E2	Positive associations between MEHP and FSH or T, MEOHP and FSH, LH or T, negative associations between MEHHP and LH, FSH or T	[82]
88 infertile men	Urinary and serum concentrations of 11 phthalate metabolites	Serum FSH, LH, T	Negative associations between FSH and MiBP and MCMHP; positive association between T and phthalates metabolites.	[83]
599 infertile men	Urinary concentrations of 8 phthalate metabolites	Serum FSH, LH, T, E2	Inverse associations between T and MiBP, FSH and MEHHP, positive relationship between E2 and MEP, %MEHP and FSH and LH	[84]
295 adult men	Urinary concentrations of phthalate metabolites	Serum FSH, LH, T, E2	Negative association between MBzP and FSH	[85]
881 healthy men	Urinary concentrations of 14 phthalate metabolites	Serum FSH, LH, T, E2	%MEHP was negatively associated with T and FSH	[86]
Male with cryptorchidism (421), hypospadias (109) or controls (425)	5cx-MEPP, 7cx-MMEHP in amniotic fluid (11–21 weeks)	INSL3, T in amniotic fluid	Negative correlations between INSL3 and cx7-MMeHP and 5cxMEPP	[87]
1066 Chinese men of reproductive age	Urinary concentrations of 14 phthalate metabolites	Serum levels of INSL3, FSH, LH, T	Negative association between INSL3 and MEHP; negative association between MBP and MiBP with T and LH	[88]
male partners of subfertile (n = 253) and fertile (n = 37) couples	11 phthalate metabolites in urine and semen	Serum levels of INSL3, FSH, LH, T, E2	Negative association between INSL3 and some urinary and seminal phthalate metabolites	[89]
case–control study of 176 men (fertile and infertile)	Urinary concentrations of 11 phthalate metabolites	Serum levels of INSL3, FSH, LH, T, E2	inverse association MMP, MiBP, MEHP, MEHP% and T; MBzP and MEHP% were negatively associated with serum INSL3 level	[90]
102 mother–child pairs	Maternal serum concentration of MEHP (23–35 weeks of gestation	Cord blood INSL3, FSH, LH, T, E2 levels	Inverse associations between maternal MEHP and INSL3 in males	[91]

Study population	EDC exposure	Matrix/ biomarker	Main results	
52 boys with cryptorchidism and 128 control boys	Cord blood BPA concentration at birth	Cord blood INSL3 levels	Higher cord blood BPA concentrations were associated with reduced cord blood INSL3 levels	[92]

T: testosterone, E2: estradiol.

Table 2.
Human biomonitoring studies addressing the relationship between EDC and hormones of HPG axis.

4.1 Hypothalamus level

4.1.1 Kisspeptin

No data are available on the impact of DDT on Kisspeptin in epidemiological studies in humans.

Interestingly, a study led on 262 mother–child pairs from China found a positive correlation between cord blood levels of BPA and *KISS1* mRNA expression in placenta tissue [60].

For phthalates, linear regression analysis showed increasing trend for kisspeptin secretion with the concentration of urinary phthalates [61].

4.1.2 GnRH

No epidemiological or experimental studies are available on the possible link between EDC levels and GnRH concentration in human. This is probably explained by the pulsatile nature of its release and the lack of dosage in clinical practice. However, many effects of EDC on GnRH were observed in rodents [93].

4.2 Pituitary level

DDT is rapidly metabolized in the body to DDE. Thus, in epidemiological studies, DDE is dosed in the blood more often than DDT. In a cohort of men of reproductive age, statistically significant positive association was found between the serum level of DDE and LH or FSH [63]. However, others studies did not reveal any association between DDT and FSH or LH levels in adult men [62, 64, 65]. In peri and postmenopausal women, inverse correlation was found between serum DDT and LH [66]. Moreover, it has been shown that maternal exposure to DDT or DDE, assayed in prenatal serum, induced a reduction of plasma LH in teenage boys, not found for FSH [67]. A study also showed that the serum levels of LH (basal level and after GnRH stimulation) was significantly higher in girls with detectable serum DDE levels than in girls with undetectable DDE [68]. This difference was not found for FSH [68].

For BPA, studies found that higher urinary BPA concentration was associated with significantly higher concentrations of serum LH in healthy young men, with or without association with FSH [69–71]. However, these results were not confirmed in others cohorts of fertile men [73]. Conversely, another study found a positive correlation between urinary BPA concentration and FSH level, without change in LH level in a cohort of infertile men [72]. In women, no association was found between urinary bisphenol A and LH or FSH levels in premenopausal women [74–76]. Moreover, no association was found in healthy children for LH and FSH [77, 78]. A modest negative correlation was found between urinary BPA concentration and peak of GnRH-stimulated FSH levels in girls with idiopathic central precocious puberty, without difference for LH levels [79].

Maternal phthalates exposure (urinary samples collected during second trimester) was not associated with serum LH level or FSH in offspring during mini-puberty in boys and girls [80]. However, positive correlations were observed between different phthalates and serum LH in prepubescent Korean children (for serum DBP or MEHP) [81], in girls with attention-deficit/hyperactivity disorder (for urinary MEP) [78] and in Chinese population (11–88 years, males and females) (for urinary MEHHP levels) [82]. In the same populations, either negative [82, 83] or no effects [78, 81] were observed on FSH level. In men, urinary phthalate metabolites were positively associated with LH and FSH levels [84] in one study while negative association between urinary phthalates concentrations and levels of FSH was found in American men (for MBzP) [85] and in Danish men (for MEHP or %MiNP) [86] without impact on LH.

Altogether, epidemiological data have linked exposure to EDC and LH and/or FSH level but evidence were often inconclusive. The inconsistent findings may partly be due to differences in the characteristics and sizes of the cohorts and to the different EDC exposure levels among studies.

4.3 Gonadal level

4.3.1 Sexual steroid hormones

Many data are already available on the effect of endocrine disruptors on the secretion of sex steroids. Recent reviews list all available studies for DDT [93], BPA [93, 94] or phthalates [93, 95–97].

4.3.2 INSL3

No data are available on the impact of DDT on INSL3 in humans epidemiological studies.

Several studies showed that INSL3 was negatively impacted by putative phthalate metabolites. The Diisononyl phthalate (DiNP) metabolite, cx7-MMeHP, and the DEHP metabolite, 5cxMEPP, showed significant negative correlations with INSL3 in amniotic fluid for weeks 11–22 [87]. Moreover, serum levels of INSL3 was negatively associated with urinary concentration of mono-2-ethylhexyl phthalate (MEHP) and MBzP among large cohorts of chinese men of reproductive age [88–90]. In adjusted models, quartiles increases in phthalates metabolites correlated with significant decreases in plasma INSL3 levels [88–90]. It has also been shown that maternal serum MEHP concentration (from 23–35 weeks of gestation) was negatively correlated with INSL3 level in cord blood mainly in boys [91].

There is also an inverse correlation between BPA level and concentration of INSL3 [92]. Indeed, in a population of 180 boys born after 34 weeks of gestation (52 cryptorchid and 128 control), cord blood levels of free BPA correlated negatively with INSL3 [92]. In this study, cord blood INSL3 level was also significantly decreased in the cryptorchid group compared with the control group [92].

Ex vivo studies on human testicular explant were performed, to study more precisely the effect of endocrine disruptors on the secretion of INSL3.

No data are available on the impact of DDT on INSL3 in humans experimental studies.

The exposure of fetal testis (8–12 weeks) to BPA at 10^{-8} M and 10^{-5} M for 72 h [98], significantly depressed the basal INSL3 production compared with control. This treatment also reduced INSL3 mRNA level by more than 20% [99]. However, BPA did not modify hCG or hLH-stimulated INSL3 production [98]. Conversely, in human adult testes, BPA increased significantly INSL3 production by Leydig cells, at a low doses (10^{-9} M) [100]. Interestingly, its analogs, Bisphenol B and Bisphenol S also increased INSL3 production at 10^{-9} and 10^{-8} M. Moreover, BADGE, another bisphenol, dose dependently increased INSL3 after 48 h of exposure. In contrast, BPE dose dependently inhibited INSL3 levels [100].

For phthalates, di-(2-ethylhexyl) phthalate (DEHP) and mono-(2-ethylhexyl) phthalate (MEHP) exposition on organo-cultured adult human testis did not affect Leydig cell INSL3 concentrations [101].

5. Conclusions

Most epidemiological and experimental studies focus on the effect of EDCs on the expression and secretion of hormones, as well as on the activity of nuclear steroid receptors. However, a few experimental studies have shown that G protein-coupled membrane receptors of the HPG axis are targets of EDCs as well. It can be pointed out that most of the studies analyzing the effects of EDCs on GPCRs of HPG axis have been performed with cell culture systems. *In vitro* models are valuable tools because they are easily manipulated. But the comparison of the effects of EDCs in wild-type and GPCRs- inactivated animal models could provide additional informations on the mode of action of these compounds.

Mechanisms of GPCR disruption by EDCs include: (1) changes in the expression; (2) interaction with transmembrane domain receptor; (3) modulation of intracellular signaling pathways.

The GPCRs of HPG axis, involved in diverse physiological functions, should be considered as possible contributors of the adverse effects of EDCs on reproduction. How their modulation by EDCs contributes to these deleterious effects should be an important field of investigations in the near future.

Acknowledgements

V.S was supported by funding from La Société Française d'Endocrinologie. MM was supported by funding from La Société Française d'Endocrinologie et de Diabétologie Pédiatrique and Novo Nordisk.

Conflict of interest

The authors declare no conflict of interest.

Author details

Valentine Suteau[1,2], Patrice Rodien[1,2,3] and Mathilde Munier[1,2,3]*

1 UMR CNRS 6015, INSERM 1083, University of Angers, France

2 Department of Endocrinology, University Hospital, Angers, France

3 Reference Center for Rare Diseases of Thyroid and Hormone Receptors, Angers, France

*Address all correspondence to: mathilde.munier@univ-angers.fr

References

[1] Diamanti-Kandarakis E, Bourguignon J-P, Giudice LC, Hauser R, Prins GS, Soto AM, et al. Endocrine-disrupting chemicals: an Endocrine Society scientific statement. Endocr Rev. 2009 Jun;30(4):293-342.

[2] Zoeller RT, Brown TR, Doan LL, Gore AC, Skakkebaek NE, Soto AM, et al. Endocrine-Disrupting Chemicals and Public Health Protection: A Statement of Principles from The Endocrine Society. Endocrinology. 2012 Sep;153(9):4097-4110.

[3] Gore AC, Chappell VA, Fenton SE, Flaws JA, Nadal A, Prins GS, et al. EDC-2: The Endocrine Society's Second Scientific Statement on Endocrine-Disrupting Chemicals. Endocr Rev. 2015 Dec;36(6):E1-150.

[4] Jiang D, Chen W-Q, Zeng X, Tang L. Dynamic Stocks and Flows Analysis of Bisphenol A (BPA) in China: 2000-2014. Environ Sci Technol. 2018 20;52(6):3706-15.

[5] Burstyn I, Martin JW, Beesoon S, Bamforth F, Li Q, Yasui Y, et al. Maternal exposure to bisphenol-A and fetal growth restriction: a case-referent study. Int J Environ Res Public Health. 2013 Dec 11;10(12):7001-7014.

[6] Carwile JL, Luu HT, Bassett LS, Driscoll DA, Yuan C, Chang JY, et al. Polycarbonate bottle use and urinary bisphenol A concentrations. Environ Health Perspect. 2009 Sep;117(9):1368-1372.

[7] Woodruff TJ, Zota AR, Schwartz JM. Environmental chemicals in pregnant women in the United States: NHANES 2003-2004. Environ Health Perspect. 2011 Jun;119(6):878-885.

[8] Radke EG, Braun JM, Meeker JD, Cooper GS. Phthalate exposure and male reproductive outcomes: A systematic review of the human epidemiological evidence. Environ Int. 2018;121(Pt 1):764-793.

[9] Hall JM, Greco CW. Perturbation of Nuclear Hormone Receptors by Endocrine Disrupting Chemicals: Mechanisms and Pathological Consequences of Exposure. Cells. 2019 19;9(1).

[10] Fredriksson R, Lagerström MC, Lundin L-G, Schiöth HB. The G-Protein-Coupled Receptors in the Human Genome Form Five Main Families. Phylogenetic Analysis, Paralogon Groups, and Fingerprints. Mol Pharmacol. 2003 Jun 1;63(6):1256-1272.

[11] Rosenbaum DM, Rasmussen SGF, Kobilka BK. The structure and function of G-protein-coupled receptors. Nature. 2009 May 21;459(7245):356-363.

[12] Sriram K, Insel PA. G Protein-Coupled Receptors as Targets for Approved Drugs: How Many Targets and How Many Drugs? Mol Pharmacol. 2018 Apr 1;93(4):251-258.

[13] Bockaert J, Philippe Pin J. Molecular tinkering of G protein-coupled receptors: an evolutionary success. EMBO J. 1999 Apr 1;18(7):1723-1729.

[14] Weis WI, Kobilka BK. The Molecular Basis of G Protein–Coupled Receptor Activation. Annu Rev Biochem. 2018 Jun 20;87:897-919.

[15] Wang W, Qiao Y, Li Z. New Insights into Modes of GPCR Activation. Trends Pharmacol Sci. 2018 Apr 1;39(4):367-386.

[16] Wong SK-F. G Protein Selectivity Is Regulated by Multiple Intracellular Regions of GPCRs. Neurosignals. 2003;12(1):1-12.

[17] Smrcka AV, Fisher I. G-protein βγ subunits as multi-functional scaffolds

and transducers in G-protein-coupled receptor signaling. Cell Mol Life Sci. 2019 Nov 1;76(22):4447-4459.

[18] Peterson YK, Luttrell LM. The Diverse Roles of Arrestin Scaffolds in G Protein–Coupled Receptor Signaling. Pharmacol Rev. 2017 Jul;69(3):256-297.

[19] Kaprara A, Huhtaniemi IT. The hypothalamus-pituitary-gonad axis: Tales of mice and men. Metabolism. 2018 Sep 1;86:3-17.

[20] Heitman LH, IJzerman AP. G protein-coupled receptors of the hypothalamic–pituitary–gonadal axis: A case for gnrh, LH, FSH, and GPR54 receptor ligands. Med Res Rev. 2008;28(6):975-1011.

[21] Young J, Xu C, Papadakis GE, Acierno JS, Maione L, Hietamäki J, et al. Clinical Management of Congenital Hypogonadotropic Hypogonadism. Endocr Rev. 2019 Apr 1;40(2):669-710.

[22] Trevisan CM, Montagna E, de Oliveira R, Christofolini DM, Barbosa CP, Crandall KA, et al. Kisspeptin/GPR54 System: What Do We Know About Its Role in Human Reproduction? Cell Physiol Biochem. 2018;49(4):1259-1276.

[23] Franssen D, Tena-Sempere M. The kisspeptin receptor: A key G-protein-coupled receptor in the control of the reproductive axis. Best Pract Res Clin Endocrinol Metab. 2018 Apr 1;32(2):107-123.

[24] Cahoreau C, Klett D, Combarnous Y. Structure–Function Relationships of Glycoprotein Hormones and Their Subunits' Ancestors. Front Endocrinol [Internet]. 2015 Feb 26 [cited 2020 Oct 13];6. Available from: https://www.ncbi.nlm.nih.gov/pmc/articles/PMC4341566/

[25] Minegishi T, Igarashi S, Nakamura K, Nakamura M, Tano M, Shinozaki H, et al. Functional expression of the recombinant human FSH receptor. J Endocrinol. 1994 May;141(2):369-375.

[26] Gudermann T, Birnbaumer M, Birnbaumer L. Evidence for dual coupling of the murine luteinizing hormone receptor to adenylyl cyclase and phosphoinositide breakdown and Ca2+ mobilization. Studies with the cloned murine luteinizing hormone receptor expressed in L cells. J Biol Chem. 1992 May 3;267(7):4479-4488.

[27] Ayoub MA, Landomiel F, Gallay N, Jégot G, Poupon A, Crépieux P, et al. Assessing Gonadotropin Receptor Function by Resonance Energy Transfer-Based Assays. Front Endocrinol [Internet]. 2015 [cited 2020 Oct 14];6. Available from: http://www.ncbi.nlm.nih.gov/pmc/articles/PMC4550792/

[28] Gloaguen P, Crépieux P, Heitzler D, Poupon A, Reiter E. Mapping the Follicle-Stimulating Hormone-Induced Signaling Networks. Front Endocrinol [Internet]. 2011 [cited 2020 Oct 14];2. Available from: http://www.ncbi.nlm.nih.gov/pmc/articles/PMC3364461/

[29] Siegel ET, Kim H-G, Nishimoto HK, Layman LC. The Molecular Basis of Impaired Follicle Stimulating Hormone Action. Reprod Sci. 2013 Mar;20(3):211-233.

[30] Casarini L, Lispi M, Longobardi S, Milosa F, Marca AL, Tagliasacchi D, et al. LH and hCG Action on the Same Receptor Results in Quantitatively and Qualitatively Different Intracellular Signalling. PLOS ONE. 2012 Oct 5;7(10):e46682.

[31] Revankar CM, Cimino DF, Sklar LA, Arterburn JB, Prossnitz ER. A transmembrane intracellular estrogen receptor mediates rapid cell signaling. Science. 2005 Mar 11;307(5715):1625-1630.

[32] Thomas P, Pang Y, Filardo EJ, Dong J. Identity of an Estrogen Membrane Receptor Coupled to a G Protein in Human Breast Cancer Cells. Endocrinology. 2005 Feb 1;146(2):624-632.

[33] Prossnitz ER, Maggiolini M. Mechanisms of estrogen signaling and gene expression via GPR30. Mol Cell Endocrinol. 2009 Sep 24;308(1-2):32-38.

[34] Bathgate R a. D, Halls ML, Westhuizen ET van der, Callander GE, Kocan M, Summers RJ. Relaxin Family Peptides and Their Receptors. Physiol Rev. 2013 Jan 1;93(1):405-480.

[35] Halls ML, Bathgate RAD, Sutton SW, Dschietzig TB, Summers RJ. International Union of Basic and Clinical Pharmacology. XCV. Recent Advances in the Understanding of the Pharmacology and Biological Roles of Relaxin Family Peptide Receptors 1-4, the Receptors for Relaxin Family Peptides. Pharmacol Rev. 2015 Jan 4;67(2):389-440.

[36] Nef S, Parada LF. Cryptorchidism in mice mutant for Insl3. Nat Genet. 1999 Jul;22(3):295-299.

[37] Zimmermann S, Steding G, Emmen JMA, Brinkmann AO, Nayernia K, Holstein AF, et al. Targeted Disruption of the Insl3 Gene Causes Bilateral Cryptorchidism. Mol Endocrinol. 1999 May 1;13(5):681-691.

[38] Ma Y, Zhang J, Zeng R, Qiao X, Cheng R, Nie Y, et al. Effects of the Dibutyl Phthalate (DBP) on the Expression and Activity of Aromatase in Human Granulosa Cell Line KGN. Ann Clin Lab Sci. 2019 Mar;49(2):175-182.

[39] Rossi M, Dimida A, Dell'anno MT, Trincavelli ML, Agretti P, Giorgi F, et al. The thyroid disruptor 1,1,1-trichloro-2,2-bis(p-chlorophenyl)-ethane appears to be an uncompetitive inverse agonist for the thyrotropin receptor. J Pharmacol Exp Ther. 2007 Jan;320(1):465-474.

[40] Younglai EV. Synergistic effects between FSH and 1,1-dichloro-2,2-bis(P-chlorophenyl)ethylene (P,P'-DDE) on human granulosa cell aromatase activity. Hum Reprod. 2004 Mar 25;19(5):1089-1093.

[41] Munier M, Grouleff J, Gourdin L, Fauchard M, Chantreau V, Henrion D, et al. In Vitro Effects of the Endocrine Disruptor p,p'DDT on Human Follitropin Receptor. Environ Health Perspect. 2016 Feb 19;

[42] Mannelli C, Szóstek AZ, Lukasik K, Carotenuto C, Ietta F, Romagnoli R, et al. Bisphenol A modulates receptivity and secretory function of human decidual cells: an in vitro study. Reprod Camb Engl. 2015 Aug;150(2):115-125.

[43] Suteau V, Briet C, Lebeault M, Gourdin L, Henrion D, Rodien P, et al. Human amniotic fluid-based exposure levels of phthalates and bisphenol A mixture reduce INSL3/RXFP2 signaling. Environ Int. 2020 May;138:105585.

[44] Castillo-Sanchez R, Ramirez-Ricardo J, Martinez-Baeza E, Cortes-Reynosa P, Candanedo-Gonzales F, Gomez R, et al. Bisphenol A induces focal adhesions assembly and activation of FAK, Src and ERK2 via GPER in MDA-MB-231 breast cancer cells. Toxicol Vitro Int J Publ Assoc BIBRA. 2020 Aug;66:104871.

[45] Bouskine A, Nebout M, Brücker-Davis F, Benahmed M, Fenichel P. Low doses of bisphenol A promote human seminoma cell proliferation by activating PKA and PKG via a membrane G-protein-coupled estrogen receptor. Environ Health Perspect. 2009 Jul;117(7):1053-1058.

[46] Thomas P, Dong J. Binding and activation of the seven-transmembrane estrogen receptor GPR30 by

environmental estrogens: a potential novel mechanism of endocrine disruption. J Steroid Biochem Mol Biol. 2006 Dec;102(1-5):175-9.

[47] Pupo M, Pisano A, Lappano R, Santolla MF, De Francesco EM, Abonante S, et al. Bisphenol A Induces Gene Expression Changes and Proliferative Effects through GPER in Breast Cancer Cells and Cancer-Associated Fibroblasts. Environ Health Perspect. 2012 Aug;120(8):1177-1182.

[48] Zhang K-S, Chen H-Q, Chen Y-S, Qiu K-F, Zheng X-B, Li G-C, et al. Bisphenol A stimulates human lung cancer cell migration via upregulation of matrix metalloproteinases by GPER/EGFR/ERK1/2 signal pathway. Biomed Pharmacother. 2014 Oct 1;68(8):1037-1043.

[49] Huang M, Huang M, Li X, Liu S, Fu L, Jiang X, et al. Bisphenol A induces apoptosis through GPER-dependent activation of the ROS/Ca2+-ASK1-JNK pathway in human granulosa cell line KGN. Ecotoxicol Environ Saf. 2021 Jan 15;208:111429.

[50] Chen X, Li L, Li H, Guan H, Dong Y, Li X, et al. Prenatal exposure to di-n-butyl phthalate disrupts the development of adult Leydig cells in male rats during puberty. Toxicology. 2017 Jul 1;386:19-27.

[51] Liu T, Li N, Zhu J, Yu G, Guo K, Zhou L, et al. Effects of di-(2-ethylhexyl) phthalate on the hypothalamus-pituitary-ovarian axis in adult female rats. Reprod Toxicol Elmsford N. 2014 Jul;46:141-147.

[52] Liu T, Jia Y, Zhou L, Wang Q, Sun D, Xu J, et al. Effects of Di-(2-ethylhexyl) Phthalate on the Hypothalamus-Uterus in Pubertal Female Rats. Int J Environ Res Public Health. 2016 12;13(11).

[53] Thal DM, Glukhova A, Sexton PM, Christopoulos A. Structural insights into G-protein-coupled receptor allostery. Nature. 2018;559(7712):45-53.

[54] Prossnitz ER, Hathaway HJ. What have we learned about GPER function in physiology and disease from knockout mice? J Steroid Biochem Mol Biol. 2015 Sep;153:114-126.

[55] Prossnitz ER, Arterburn JB. International Union of Basic and Clinical Pharmacology. XCVII. G Protein–Coupled Estrogen Receptor and Its Pharmacologic Modulators. Pharmacol Rev. 2015 Jul;67(3):505-540.

[56] Yang W, Tan W, Zheng J, Zhang B, Li H, Li X. MEHP promotes the proliferation of cervical cancer via GPER mediated activation of Akt. Eur J Pharmacol. 2018 Apr 5;824:11-16.

[57] Castillo Sanchez R, Gomez R, Perez Salazar E. Bisphenol A Induces Migration through a GPER-, FAK-, Src-, and ERK2-Dependent Pathway in MDA-MB-231 Breast Cancer Cells. Chem Res Toxicol. 2016 Mar 21;29(3):285-295.

[58] Cao L-Y, Ren X-M, Li C-H, Zhang J, Qin W-P, Yang Y, et al. Bisphenol AF and Bisphenol B Exert Higher Estrogenic Effects than Bisphenol A via G Protein-Coupled Estrogen Receptor Pathway. Environ Sci Technol. 2017 Oct 3;51(19):11423-11430.

[59] Lei B, Sun S, Zhang X, Feng C, Xu J, Wen Y, et al. Bisphenol AF exerts estrogenic activity in MCF-7 cells through activation of Erk and PI3K/Akt signals via GPER signaling pathway. Chemosphere. 2019 Apr;220:362-370.

[60] Xu X, Chiung YM, Lu F, Qiu S, Ji M, Huo X. Associations of cadmium, bisphenol A and polychlorinated biphenyl co-exposure in utero with placental gene expression and neonatal outcomes. Reprod Toxicol. 2015 Apr 1;52:62-70.

[61] Chen C-Y, Chou Y-Y, Wu Y-M, Lin C-C, Lin S-J, Lee C-C. Phthalates may promote female puberty by increasing kisspeptin activity. Hum Reprod. 2013 Oct 1;28(10):2765-2773.

[62] Bornman M, Delport R, Farías P, Aneck-Hahn N, Patrick S, Millar RP, et al. Alterations in male reproductive hormones in relation to environmental DDT exposure. Environ Int. 2018 Apr 1;113:281-289.

[63] Giwercman Aleksander, Rignell-Hydbom Anna, Toft Gunnar, Rylander Lars, Hagmar Lars, Lindh Christian, et al. Reproductive Hormone Levels in Men Exposed to Persistent Organohalogen Pollutants: A Study of Inuit and Three European Cohorts. Environ Health Perspect. 2006 Sep 1;114(9):1348-1353.

[64] Asawasinsopon R, Prapamontol T, Prakobvitayakit O, Vaneesorn Y, Mangklabruks A, Hock B. Plasma levels of DDT and their association with reproductive hormones in adult men from northern Thailand. Sci Total Environ. 2006 Feb 15;355(1):98-105.

[65] Cocco P, Loviselli A, Fadda D, Ibba A, Melis M, Oppo A, et al. Serum sex hormones in men occupationally exposed to dichloro-diphenyl-trichloro ethane (DDT) as young adults. J Endocrinol. 2004 Sep 1;182(3):391-397.

[66] Freire C, Koifman RJ, Sarcinelli PN, Rosa ACS, Clapauch R, Koifman S. Association between serum levels of organochlorine pesticides and sex hormones in adults living in a heavily contaminated area in Brazil. Int J Hyg Environ Health. 2014 Mar 1;217(2):370-378.

[67] Eskenazi B, Rauch SA, Tenerelli R, Huen K, Holland NT, Lustig RH, et al. In utero and childhood DDT, DDE, PBDE and PCBs exposure and sex hormones in adolescent boys: The CHAMACOS study. Int J Hyg Environ Health. 2017 Apr 1;220(2, Part B):364-72.

[68] Ozen S, Darcan S, Bayindir P, Karasulu E, Simsek DG, Gurler T. Effects of pesticides used in agriculture on the development of precocious puberty. Environ Monit Assess. 2012 Jul 1;184(7):4223-4232.

[69] Lassen TH, Frederiksen H, Jensen TK, Petersen JH, Joensen UN, Main KM, et al. Urinary Bisphenol A Levels in Young Men: Association with Reproductive Hormones and Semen Quality. Environ Health Perspect. 2014 May;122(5):478.

[70] Adoamnei E, Mendiola J, Vela-Soria F, Fernández MF, Olea N, Jørgensen N, et al. Urinary bisphenol A concentrations are associated with reproductive parameters in young men. Environ Res. 2018 Feb 1;161:122-128.

[71] Liang H, Xu W, Chen J, Shi H, Zhu J, Liu X, et al. The Association between Exposure to Environmental Bisphenol A and Gonadotropic Hormone Levels among Men. PLOS ONE. 2017 Jan 13;12(1):e0169217.

[72] Meeker JD, Calafat AM, Hauser R. Urinary Bisphenol A Concentrations in Relation to Serum Thyroid and Reproductive Hormone Levels in Men from an Infertility Clinic. Environ Sci Technol. 2010 Feb 15;44(4):1458.

[73] Hart RJ, Doherty DA, Keelan JA, Minaee NS, Thorstensen EB, Dickinson JE, et al. The impact of antenatal Bisphenol A exposure on male reproductive function at 20-22 years of age. Reprod Biomed Online. 2018 Mar 1;36(3):340-347.

[74] Li C, Cao M, Qi T, Ye X, Ma L, Pan W, et al. The association of bisphenol A exposure with premature ovarian insufficiency: a case–control study. Climacteric. 2020 Jul 16;0(0):1-6.

[75] Miao M, Yuan W, Yang F, Liang H, Zhou Z, Li R, et al. Associations between Bisphenol A Exposure and

Reproductive Hormones among Female Workers. Int J Environ Res Public Health. 2015 Oct;12(10):13240.

[76] Pollack AZ, Mumford SL, Krall JR, Carmichael AE, Sjaarda LA, Perkins NJ, et al. Exposure to bisphenol A, chlorophenols, benzophenones, and parabens in relation to reproductive hormones in healthy women: A chemical mixture approach. Environ Int. 2018 Nov;120:137.

[77] Mustieles V, Ocón-Hernandez O, Mínguez-Alarcón L, Dávila-Arias C, Pérez-Lobato R, Calvente I, et al. Bisphenol A and reproductive hormones and cortisol in peripubertal boys: The INMA-Granada cohort. Sci Total Environ. 2018 Mar 15;618:1046-1053.

[78] Tsai C-S, Chou W-J, Lee S-Y, Lee M-J, Chou M-C, Wang L-J. Phthalates, Para-Hydroxybenzoic Acids, Bisphenol-A, and Gonadal Hormones' Effects on Susceptibility to Attention-Deficit/Hyperactivity Disorder. Toxics. 2020 Sep;8(3):57.

[79] Chen Y, Wang Y, Ding G, Tian Y, Zhou Z, Wang X, et al. Association between bisphenol a exposure and idiopathic central precocious puberty (ICPP) among school-aged girls in Shanghai, China. Environ Int. 2018 Jun 1;115:410-416.

[80] Muerköster A-P, Frederiksen H, Juul A, Andersson A-M, Jensen RC, Glintborg D, et al. Maternal phthalate exposure associated with decreased testosterone/LH ratio in male offspring during mini-puberty. Odense Child Cohort. Environ Int. 2020 Nov 1;144:106025.

[81] Hyun Kim D, Min Choi S, Soo Lim D, Roh T, Jun Kwack S, Yoon S, et al. Risk assessment of endocrine disrupting phthalates and hormonal alterations in children and adolescents. J Toxicol Environ Health A. 2018;81(21):1150-1164.

[82] Zhang J, Yin W, Li P, Hu C, Wang L, Li T, et al. Interaction between diet- and exercise-lifestyle and phthalates exposure on sex hormone levels. J Hazard Mater. 2019 May 5;369:290-298.

[83] Wang B, Qin X, Xiao N, Yao Y, Duan Y, Cui X, et al. Phthalate exposure and semen quality in infertile male population from Tianjin, China: Associations and potential mediation by reproductive hormones. Sci Total Environ. 2020 Nov 20;744:140673.

[84] Al-Saleh I, Coskun S, Al-Doush I, Al-Rajudi T, Abduljabbar M, Al-Rouqi R, et al. The relationships between urinary phthalate metabolites, reproductive hormones and semen parameters in men attending in vitro fertilization clinic. Sci Total Environ. 2019 Mar 25;658:982-995.

[85] Duty SM, Calafat AM, Silva MJ, Ryan L, Hauser R. Phthalate exposure and reproductive hormones in adult men. Hum Reprod. 2005 Mar 1;20(3):604-610.

[86] Joensen UN, Frederiksen H, Jensen MB, Lauritsen MP, Olesen IA, Lassen TH, et al. Phthalate Excretion Pattern and Testicular Function: A Study of 881 Healthy Danish Men. Environ Health Perspect. 2012 Oct;120(10):1397-1403

[87] Anand-Ivell R, Cohen A, Nørgaard-Pedersen B, Jönsson BAG, Bonde J-P, Hougaard DM, et al. Amniotic Fluid INSL3 Measured During the Critical Time Window in Human Pregnancy Relates to Cryptorchidism, Hypospadias, and Phthalate Load: A Large Case–Control Study. Front Physiol [Internet]. 2018 Apr 24 [cited 2020 Oct 6];9. Available from: https://www.ncbi.nlm.nih.gov/pmc/articles/PMC5928321/

[88] Pan Y, Jing J, Dong F, Yao Q, Zhang W, Zhang H, et al. Association between phthalate metabolites and biomarkers of reproductive function in

1066 Chinese men of reproductive age. J Hazard Mater. 2015 Dec 30;300:729-736.

[89] Chang W-H, Wu M-H, Pan H-A, Guo P-L, Lee C-C. Semen quality and insulin-like factor 3: Associations with urinary and seminal levels of phthalate metabolites in adult males. Chemosphere. 2017 Apr;173:594-602.

[90] Chang W-H, Li S-S, Wu M-H, Pan H-A, Lee C-C. Phthalates might interfere with testicular function by reducing testosterone and insulin-like factor 3 levels. Hum Reprod. 2015 Nov 1;30(11):2658-2670.

[91] Araki A, Mitsui T, Miyashita C, Nakajima T, Naito H, Ito S, et al. Association between Maternal Exposure to di(2-ethylhexyl) Phthalate and Reproductive Hormone Levels in Fetal Blood: The Hokkaido Study on Environment and Children's Health. PLOS ONE. 2014 Oct 8;9(10):e109039.

[92] Chevalier N, Brucker-Davis F, Lahlou N, Coquillard P, Pugeat M, Pacini P, et al. A negative correlation between insulin-like peptide 3 and bisphenol A in human cord blood suggests an effect of endocrine disruptors on testicular descent during fetal development. Hum Reprod. 2015 Jan 2;30(2):447-453.

[93] Graceli JB, Dettogni RS, Merlo E, Niño O, da Costa CS, Zanol JF, et al. The impact of endocrine-disrupting chemical exposure in the mammalian hypothalamic-pituitary axis. Mol Cell Endocrinol. 2020 Aug 22;518:110997.

[94] Mustieles V, D'Cruz SC, Couderq S, Rodríguez-Carrillo A, Fini J-B, Hofer T, et al. Bisphenol A and its analogues: A comprehensive review to identify and prioritize effect biomarkers for human biomonitoring. Environ Int. 2020 Nov 1;144:105811.

[95] Pallotti F, Pelloni M, Gianfrilli D, Lenzi A, Lombardo F, Paoli D. Mechanisms of Testicular Disruption from Exposure to Bisphenol A and Phtalates. J Clin Med [Internet]. 2020 Feb 8 [cited 2020 Nov 12];9(2). Available from: https://www.ncbi.nlm.nih.gov/pmc/articles/PMC7074154/

[96] Radke EG, Glenn BS, Braun JM, Cooper GS. Phthalate exposure and female reproductive and developmental outcomes: a systematic review of the human epidemiological evidence. Environ Int. 2019 Sep 1;130:104580.

[97] Radke EG, Braun JM, Meeker JD, Cooper GS. Phthalate exposure and male reproductive outcomes: A systematic review of the human epidemiological evidence. Environ Int. 2018 Dec 1;121:764-793.

[98] Maamar MB, Lesné L, Desdoits-Lethimonier C, Coiffec I, Lassurguère J, Lavoué V, et al. An Investigation of the Endocrine-Disruptive Effects of Bisphenol A in Human and Rat Fetal Testes. PLoS ONE [Internet]. 2015 Feb 23 [cited 2017 Jul 10];10(2). Available from: http://www.ncbi.nlm.nih.gov/pmc/articles/PMC4338204/

[99] N'Tumba-Byn T, Moison D, Lacroix M, Lecureuil C, Lesage L, Prud'homme SM, et al. Differential Effects of Bisphenol A and Diethylstilbestrol on Human, Rat and Mouse Fetal Leydig Cell Function. PLoS ONE [Internet]. 2012 Dec 17 [cited 2017 Jul 10];7(12). Available from: http://www.ncbi.nlm.nih.gov/pmc/articles/PMC3524173/

[100] Desdoits-Lethimonier C, Lesné L, Gaudriault P, Zalko D, Antignac JP, Deceuninck Y, et al. Parallel assessment of the effects of bisphenol A and several of its analogs on the adult human testis. Hum Reprod. 2017 Jul 1;32(7):1465-1473.

[101] Desdoits-Lethimonier C, Albert O, Le Bizec B, Perdu E, Zalko D, Courant F, et al. Human testis steroidogenesis is inhibited by phthalates. Hum Reprod. 2012 May 1;27(5):1451-1459.

Chapter 2

Effect of Endocrine Disrupting Chemicals on HPG Axis: A Reproductive Endocrine Homeostasis

Priya Gupta, Archisman Mahapatra, Anjali Suman and Rahul Kumar Singh

Abstract

The hypothalamic–pituitary-gonadal (HPG) axis plays a crucial and integrative role in the mammalian endocrine regulation to maintain homeostasis. The HPG axis is primarily responsible for governing all the hormonal events related to reproductive activity. Endocrine-disrupting chemicals (EDCs) comprise a diverse group of naturally occurring and synthetic compounds that mimic and interfere with the endogenous chemical hormones. Epidemiological investigations have shown increasing evidence of altered development and detrimental effects on reproductive health during the past 50 years associated with endocrine disruptors affecting the HPG axis. The pleiotropic harmful effects of EDCs act through hormone-dependent downstream signaling pathways responsible for gonad development either through direct interaction with steroid hormone receptor or via epigenetic regulation. Hence, this chapter summarizes the biological plausibility of EDCs exposure and elucidates the mechanism of action underlying EDCs affecting the regulatory circuits of the mammalian HPG axis and reproductive function.

Keywords: endocrine disrupting chemicals, hypothalmic-pituitary-gonadal axis, reproduction, epigenetic, polycystic ovarian syndrome

1. Introduction

In the past decade, endocrine disruptor chemicals (EDCs) in human pathophysiology have gained much more attention due to their ability to affect development and reproduction in humans and wildlife. In accordance with the US Environmental Protection Agency (EPA), EDCs can be defined as 'exogenous agents that disrupt the hormone homeostasis by interfering with the synthesis, secretion, transport, metabolism, receptor binding or elimination of endogenous hormone [1–6]. EDCs comprise mainly heterogeneous compounds, including synthetic (chemical) and natural (plant products such as isoflavones) responsible for disrupting the hormone system. Endocrine disruptors may be found easily in almost every product used in our daily life, including detergents, plastic bottles, food, toys, pesticides, insecticides, and flame retardants. The criteria proposed by the European Commission for being in the process of defining any compound as EDCs should at least exhibit three

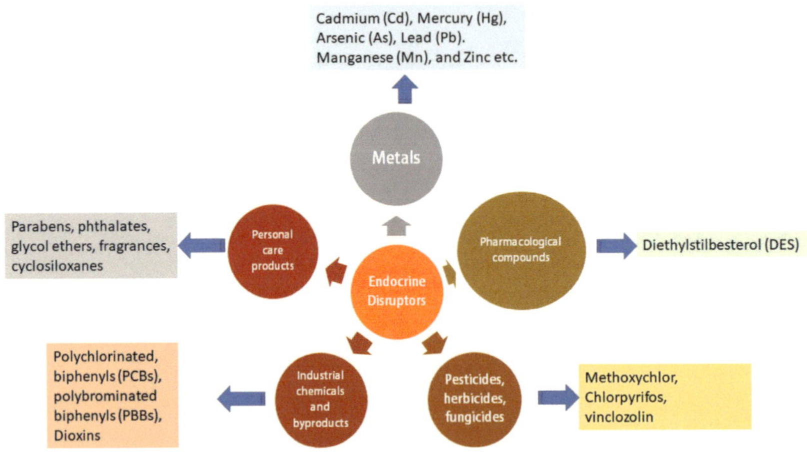

Figure 1.
Sources and examples of EDCs.

characters: (1) an endocrine activity, (2) an adverse or deleterious endocrine mediated effect in the exposed subject or its progeny or subpopulations (3) a plausible cause-effect relationship between the two [7, 8]. Most of the EDCs interfere with the endocrine system by binding the hormonal receptor or regulating genomic expression. Increasing evidence has documented that the highest risk is posed during early and postnatal development while forming organ and neural systems [9]. Sometimes, epigenetic changes (DNA methylation or acetylation) or histone modifications are also involved in endocrine disruption [10].

EDCs are highly heterogeneous and can be classified based on their origin: Industrial and household chemicals (dioxins, phthalates, polychlorinated biphenyls (PCBs), alkylphenols, plasticizers, fire retardants), agricultural (insecticides, pesticides, herbicides, fungicides, phytoestrogens), residential {bisphenol A (BPA), polybrominated biphenyls (PBBs), phthalates} and some pharmaceuticals agents {parabens, diethylstilbestrol (DES)} [3, 5, 11]. Heavy metals such as lead, mercury, cadmium, and arsenic are also included in the EDCs long list (**Figure 1**) [10, 12]. According to the Stockholm Convention (2001), both production and usage of persistent organic pollutants (POPs) was restricted [13]. Guidelines for a list of chemicals were developed to store and eliminate them, which was happened in 2008 and 2014 [14]. Initially, almost twelve POPs were designated as "dirty dozen" due to their severe adverse effects on humans and the ecosystem. Hence, their production and use were banned. The dirty dozen included industrial chemicals, pesticides, and by-products such as aldrin, chlordane, dieldrin, endrin, dichlorodiphenyltrichloroethane (DDT), heptachlor, mirex, toxaphene, PCBs, hexachlorobenzene, polychlorinated dibenzo-p-dioxins, and polychlorinated dibenzofurans [9].

2. Human exposure and route of entry of EDCs

Endocrine-disrupting chemicals may exhibit various exposure routes to enter the human body. Generally, inhalation (e.g., Plasticizers), dietary intake (e.g., Foods), dermal absorption (e.g., Cosmetics), and embryonic exposure (e.g., Transfer from mother) represent the main exposure pathways (**Figure 2**) [5, 15]. Following any of these pathways, EDCs may enter the food chain and accumulate in different tissues [16]. Mostly EDCs are highly lipophilic in nature and hence accumulate in the adipose tissue having a long half-life. These aforementioned

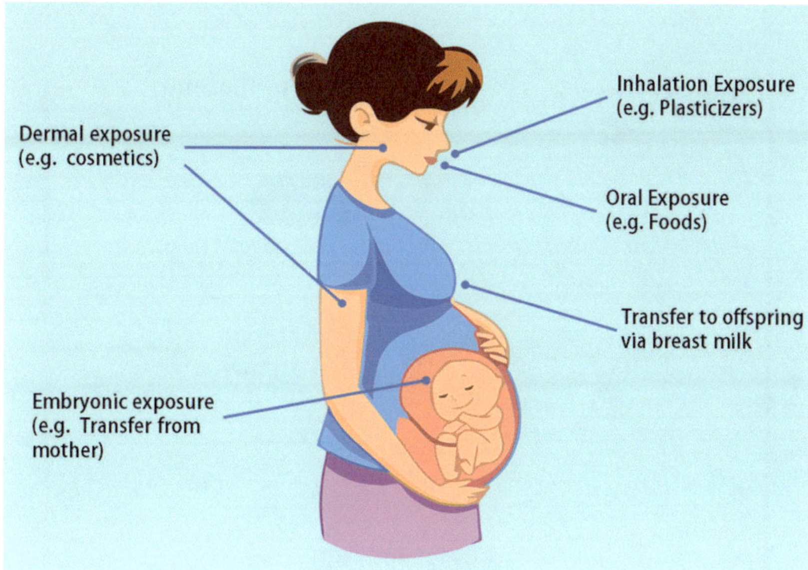

Figure 2.
Route of entries of EDCs.

features explain the exact reasons for being the accumulation of EDCs for years in the adipose tissue. Humans and other top predators are at the top of the food chain. Hence, due to bioaccumulation and biomagnification, they may store many EDCs, ultimately leading to various adverse consequences. Even lifelong exposure or fetal or neonatal stage exposure may bring about cumulative or additive or synergic effects. Therefore, the timing of exposure is of utmost importance in evaluating adverse effects on the endocrine system.

Endocrine disruptors such as dioxins, PCBs, perfluorinated compounds, and DDT are commonly found in pesticide-contaminated soil or groundwater or industrial waste quickly enter the human body via oral consumption of food or water. Some of the commonly used EDCs (DDT, vinclozolin, pyrethroids, chlorpyrifos) in households, agriculture, or public disease vector control may come in contact with human skin or through inhalation. In addition to this, cosmetics, personal care products, sunscreens, medications (triclosan, paraben, phthalates) that we apply on our skin are also responsible for their uptake into our body [17]. Professional workers using fungicides, pesticides, and chemicals are most prone and at high risk of EDCs exposure.

3. HPG axis: the central regulator

The mammalian reproductive cycles are mainly controlled by an intricate play between hypothalamus pituitary and gonads [18]. The hypothalamic Gonadotropin-Releasing Hormone (GnRH) neurons regulate reproductive functions in all vertebrates. The hypothalamic–pituitary-gonadal (HPG) axis plays a crucial role in the normal development of the reproductive system by controlling the ovarian as well as uterine cycles in females and also spermatogenesis in males [18, 19]. In response to GnRH release from the hypothalamus, pituitary gonadotropic cells synthesize and release Luteinizing Hormone (LH) and Follicle-Stimulating Hormone (FSH), which travel via the bloodstream to the target organs. LH and FSH are essential as regulators of both ovarian and testicular function. In males, LH stimulates

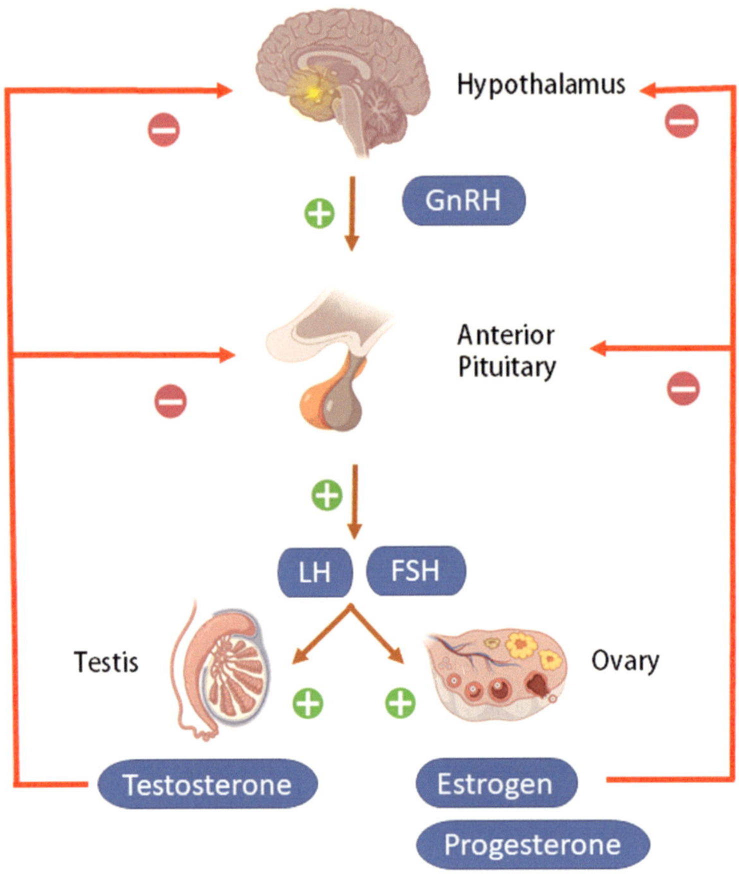

Figure 3.
Regulation of HPG axis.

testicular Leydig cells to synthesize and secrete testosterone, which in turn maintains spermatogenesis in Sertoli cells through its paracrine action and exerts sexual and anabolic actions. While FSH acts on Sertoli cells to produce androgen-binding protein, which is critical for spermatogenesis initiation and ultimately augments sperm production [20]. In females, the production of GnRH, LH, and FSH via the HPG axis are similar, but the actions of these hormones are different. LH and FSH exert their function on the ovaries to promote follicular maturation, ovulation, corpus luteum development, and estrogen and progesterone production [21, 22]. These hormones also have a role in regulating the uterine (menstrual) cycle to prepare for ovulation and embryo implantation [23]. These gonadal steroid hormones secreted by ovaries and testis can inhibit GnRH's hypothalamic synthesis via a feedback loop, hence playing a vital role in regulating reproductive function. In most mammals, 17β- Estradiol, testosterone, and progesterone are the primary estrogen, androgen, and progestin, respectively, and each of their receptors are expressed abundantly in the hypothalamus (**Figure 3**) [24].

4. Molecular mechanisms of EDCs

It is widely known that EDCs molecule, either natural or synthetic, follows the classical mechanism of action to mimic or interfere with the action of an endocrine regulated network of vertebrates. This interference can happen through different mechanisms, either through genomic or non-genomic actions. So before understanding the mechanism of endocrine disruption, we must have a clear picture of the endocrine system that relies on the synthesis and release of hormones from various endocrine glands and its transport via the bloodstream to the required distant cells and tissues [25]. This process involves complex interacting signaling pathways and hormone receptors to control normal body function. Estrogen receptors (ERs) regulate the transcription of their target genes via multiple pathways, either directly or indirectly. Any changes in ER signaling may lead to adverse consequences such as hormone-dependent cancer, abnormal fetal growth and development, altered metabolism, and sometimes impaired fertility. Although the effect of EDCs is not limited to only the ligand-dependent ER signaling pathway, it is the best-studied of ER targeted endocrine disruption. ER in response to ligand signals through both genomic as well as a non-genomic pathway. Briefly, ER mediates its signal in the genomic pathway by binding directly to estrogen-responsive elements (ERE) or indirectly through coactivators such as SP-1 or AP-1. Although the best well-studied nuclear receptor cofactors belong to the p160 family of coactivators (e.g., SRC-1, SRC-2, and SRC-3) but the cofactor complex that mediates ER signaling is more complicated.

The non-genomic pathway has a rapid response as within minutes of ligand binding, signal transduction occurs. During estrogen ligand, a G-protein coupled receptor (GPCR-30) activates and mediates the signal independent of ERs and stimulates cAMP production, fluctuates intracellular calcium, or lead to MAPK or PI3K signaling cascades events. BPA and DES are extensively studied EDCs, which also induce rapid estrogen signaling via the non-genomic pathway (**Figure 4**).

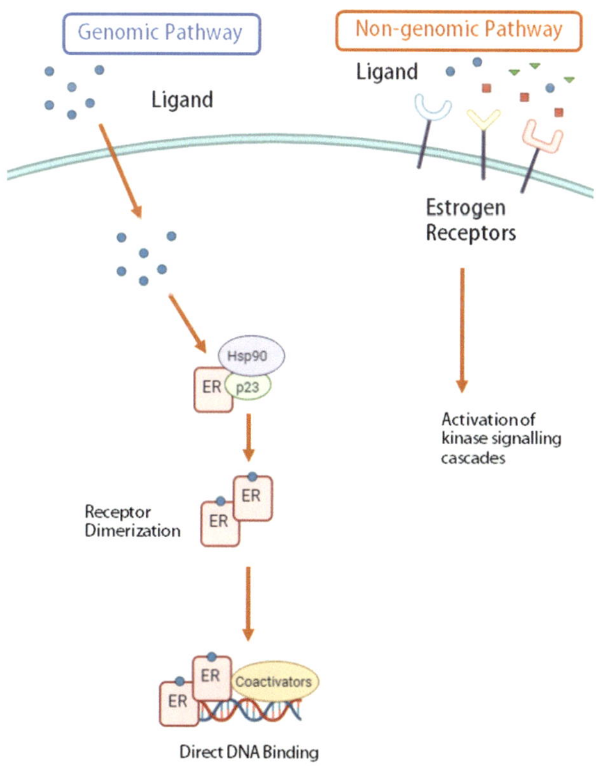

Figure 4.
Genomic and non-genomic pathway of estrogen signaling.

Steroid hormones are a group of lipophilic molecules that regulate a wide variety of physiological functions starting from fetal life to adulthood [26]. All these steroid hormones are biosynthesized from cholesterol, including glucocorticoids, mineralocorticoids, progestin, estrogen, and androgen, regulating sexual and reproductive development. Steroidogenic enzymes involved in the steroid hormone biosynthesis pathway are considered as the crucial targets for EDCs action. For example, Researches have demonstrated that exposure of Nonylphenol (NP) concentration 10^{-4} to 10^{-1} M at several ages with multiple rat generations (N = 3-4 per group) can decrease P450scc activity in testes [27]. Phthalates exposure, which consists of a particular class of pesticides, inhibits testosterone synthesis in Leydig cells due to direct CYP17 inhibition and hence exerts anti-androgenic effects [28]. Furthermore, BPA of different concentrations (10^{-8} to 10^{-4} M) have been shown to inhibit the enzymatic activity of 3β-HSD, CYP17A1, and 17β-HSD3 in a dose-dependent manner in both human and rat testicular microsomes [29]. EDCs exposure also inhibits the activity of 5-α reductase, which is one of the main enzymes involved in dihydrotestosterone production from testosterone and hence in the regulation of masculinization of the external genitalia and the prostrate [30].

Aromatase (cyp19a) is known as the potential target action of EDC, and any modulation in its expression and function alters the estrogen production rate and hence disrupts the estrogen-dependent process [31]. A study suggested that BPA exposure in rat testis R2C Leydig cells stimulate aromatase activity and is correlated with upregulation in COX-2 in R2C cells [32].

In addition to steroidogenic enzymes and hormone metabolism, EDCs are also known to affect hormone-related receptor and their expression. EDCs, due to their similarity in structural features with the endogenous estrogen hormones, bind easily with the estrogen receptors and thus modify estrogen-responsive gene expression. EDCs that display binding with ERs include industrial bisphenolics, pharmaceutical chemicals, phytoestrogens, and organochlorine pesticides. Methoxychlor (MTX) and DDT are examples of organochlorine pesticides that exhibit estrogenic activity through binding with ERα and ERβ ligand-binding domains [33]. Thus, as reported, both pesticides adversely affect the female reproductive trait by impairing normal follicle development and stimulating uterine proliferation [34]. The insecticide endosulfan has a similar estrogenic activity that causes ovarian regression in both in vitro and in vivo studies [35]. Endosulfan competes with estradiol for interacting with the estrogen receptor but with lower affinity and, in turn, affects sex-specific gene expression [36]. Endosulfan can also affect the male reproductive system by decreasing the gene expression of testis-related transcription factors (sox9a and wt1) [37]. BPA possesses a binding affinity for ERs subtypes (ERα and ERβ) and is categorized as a prototypical non-steroidal ER [38].

It is also important to note that EDCs exhibit multiple hormone-binding actions regardless of their binding to hormonal receptors. For instance, DDT is an agonist for the estrogen receptor, but one of the metabolites of DDT shows anti-androgenic activity [39]. Similarly, BPA shows estrogenic and androgenic activity but exhibits an antagonist nature for thyroid hormone [40, 41].

5. Effect of EDCs on female reproductive system

The female reproductive system's development is credited to folliculogenesis, where adverse biological effects of EDCs can be observed. The primordial follicles finally become primary, pre-antral, and the antral follicle. Environmental toxicants such as BPA, MTX, and phthalates may interfere at any developmental stage of the aforementioned antral follicle growth and hinder the reproduction, sometimes causing infertility. BPA exposure during in-vitro studies has been shown to inhibit mouse antral follicle development [42]. Follicle growth is dependent on the proliferation of theca and granulosa cells [43].

Estrogens are well-known as the gatekeepers of the female reproductive system. The sudden increase during puberty opens the gate to enter the reproductive life, and at menopause, the gate gets closed due to their decreased level. Thus, the environmental chemicals that behave as agonists or antagonists to estrogen hormone may play a role in precocious puberty, polycystic ovary syndrome, delay in menopause, and premature ovarian failure [44]. Increased growth of the endometrium and breast cancer are some of the unwanted side effects in females that can also occur due to EDCs exposure.

5.1 Puberty and breast development

The growing evidence of EDCs affecting puberty or early breast development in the female has dramatically increased. It has been observed from the studies that the age of menarche has been decreased from 16-17 years to less than 13 years [5]. The increased estrogen-to-androgen ratio due to overexpression of aromatase activity has been shown to cause early or premature breast development and sometimes gynecomastia in boys [45, 46].

5.2 Breast cancer

Breast cancer is a multifactorial disease [47] and mainly results from time-related complex interactions between internal and external factors [48]. Although endogenous estrogen has a role in breast tumor genesis, but estrogen-mimicking exogenous EDCs such as PCBs, BPA, DES, and phthalates have substantial impacts on breast development during the perinatal period and also on carcinogenesis in adults [48]. Studies have reported that women with prenatal exposure to DES, a synthetic estrogen, have an increased risk of breast cancer in their later age (≥40 years) [49]. Perinatal BPA exposure at environmentally relevant concentration alters breast development in both outbred mice and rats. The mode of action of estrogen-mimicking EDCs is two-fold; firstly, their action is on the proliferation of stromal cells and, secondly, concerned with epigenetic mechanisms [50]. EDCs affect the stromal cells by interfering with the estrogen signal pathway. HOXB9 is a homeobox-containing gene that plays a vital role in mammary gland development and is associated with breast cancer. Reports have shown that BPA competes with ER and leads to activation of this gene through histone modification and acetylation [50].

5.3 Uterine disease

Endometriosis and uterine fibroids are the most common female reproductive disorders, having an estimated combined incidence of up to 70% of women. Due to their cryptic nature, many women with either endometriosis or fibroids may remain asymptomatic or undiagnosed and are more likely caused due to environmental endocrine-active compounds. For instance, non-human primates exposed to environmental contaminant TCDD (dioxin) have a higher endometriosis rate. The onset of fibroids occurs mainly after puberty, and this benign uterine tumor regresses after menopause. Fibroids are found to be more sensitive to the estrogen effect [51]. Hence, due to its dependency on estrogen for its growth, the role of environmental estrogen-mimicking EDCs in fibroid disease should be considered.

Several reports have documented that developmental exposure to EDCs such as MTX, PCBs, DDT, DES have been implicated in the development of uterine fibroid disease [52].

5.4 Primary ovarian failure (POF)

About 1% of the female population under 40 years of age suffers from POF, leading to other comorbidities related to reproductive disorder or early menopause [53]. The possible mechanism of POF development includes premature activation of the follicle, blockage of follicle maturation, and acceleration of apoptosis. Several cases of POF have been reported, and EDCs might have some association with its occurrence. Many EDCs are related to multi-oocyte follicles (MOF) mediated by EDCs-induced ERβ agonist action. Administration of BPA (0.1-1,000 μg/kg) to pregnant mice between the critical periods of differentiation (9th-16th day), ovarian cysts appeared in adulthood, which was significantly more in number in the group that received 1 μg/kg BPA [54]. Paraben is another example of EDC that affects folliculogenesis by stimulating anti-mullerian hormone (AMH) mRNA expression and inhibits the early stage of ovarian follicle in newborn rats [44]. Similarly, MTX inhibits folliculogenesis and increases AMH expression in the pre-antral and early-antral follicles [55]. Recent studies have demonstrated that neonatal exposure of DES (3 μg/kg) induces MOF [56].

5.5 Menstrual irregularity

Studies have shown that fetal and neonatal exposure to EDCs exposure in humans may interfere with hormonal regulation and result in irregular or long cycles of the menstrual cycle [57]. The irregularities in the menstrual cycle may ultimately reduce fecundity. In-utero exposure to estrogenic compounds such as phytoestrogens or BPA in an animal model such as adult mice increases estrous cycle duration. In comparison, perinatal exposure to BPA results in early suspension and irregular cyclic activity [58] that are likely due to a change in LH secretion's hypothalamic control and ovulation [59].

5.6 Polycystic ovarian syndrome (PCOS)

This disease is a more prevalent endocrine disorder in women, characterized by anovulation and hyperandrogenism. This syndrome is associated with a higher

Reference	Chemicals	Organism	Results
[5]	EDCs	Human	Decreased age of menarche
[54]	BPA	Mice	Induces PCOS
[44]	Paraben	Rats	Inhibit early stage of ovarian follicle
[55]	MTX	Rats	Increase the expression of AMH in the pre-antral and early-antral follicles
[56]	DES	Mice	Induces MOF
[57]	PBD, PCB	Human	Irregular menstrual cycle
[58]	BPA	Human	Irregular menstrual cycle
[60]	BPA	Human	Development of PCOS

Table 1.
A summary of the remarkable studies on effects of EDCs on female reproductive systems.

prevalence of obesity, insulin resistance, and other metabolic comorbidities. However, this disease's pathogenesis is still not exact, but evidence shows that genetic and environmental factors such as EDCs may contribute to PCOS's clinical development. BPA, a well-known estrogenic and androgenic endocrine disruptor, acts differently to interfere in reproductive functions. In vitro studies have shown that BPA exposure in rat ovarian thecal interstitial cells increases testosterone synthesis.

In contrast, in male rats, BPA competes with androgens to bind on sex hormone-binding globulin (SHBG), increasing serum-free androgen level. BPA exposure during neonatal conditions could lead to PCOS development. Besides, the estrogenic effect of environmental contaminant BPA enhances the risk of hypertension, type2 diabetes, and dyslipidemia (**Table 1**) [60].

6. Effect of EDCs on male reproductive system

A large number of studies reported the toxic effects of environmental contaminants on male reproductive health. Numerous EDCs present in our environment may have a causative role in testicular dysgenesis syndrome (TDS) in humans. Impaired spermatogenesis, decrease in semen quality, sperm anomalies, hypospadias, ectopic testes, cryptorchidism, and testicular cancer are important risk factors responsible for the symptoms of developmental disorder, TDS and ultimately causing male infertility. During the normal condition, a functional hormonal feedback loop regulates and ensures proper homeostasis. Sometimes, at the time of sexual development, exposure to certain chemicals may disrupt this tightly-regulated hormonal balance. Even short-term exposures can also have adverse effects and may cause infertility [61].

6.1 Semen and sperm quality

Semen parameters are used to measure sperm quality and are sometimes considered indicators of compromised male fertility [62]. Recently, the adverse health effects of the male reproductive system, especially due to BPA's estrogenic property, have attracted much more attention. BPA is well-known as a testicular toxicant in animal models as it results in decreased sperm quality and motility, oxidative stress increases, and alters steroidogenesis [12]. Few studies were done in occupationally exposed men, and infertile men have also reported a negative correlation between semen quality and urinary BPA levels. The underlying mechanism may be related to increased oxidative stress and disruption in the steroidogenesis pathway [63].

Functional anomalies of sperm may play a crucial role in male infertility. As reported, in comparison with fertile controls, infertile men have higher seminal reactive oxygen species (ROS) levels; hence studies have suggested ROS might have some role in male infertility. Sperm cells do not contain any cytoplasmic defense enzymes that can serve as ROS scavengers. Therefore, a change in lipid peroxidation (LPO) impairs the plasma membrane fluidity and integrity and ultimately leading to loss of sperm function and movement. Exposure to carbaryl causes low LPO concentrations with an increase in ROS and hence may be associated with altered semen quality, especially sperm motility [64].

Furthermore, BPA was also associated with DNA damage, lower sperm count, abnormal sperm morphology, and motion [65]. Regarding the hormonal level, BPA caused higher FSH, lower inhibin B level, and a lower estradiol-to-testosterone ratio [65]. In a study comprising 375 fertile men, BPA was further associated with decreased free androgen index and higher testosterone level [66].

Reference	Chemicals	Organism	Results
[42]	BPA	Human	Decreased sperm quality and motility, altered steroidogenesis
[63]	BPA	Rat	Disrupted steroidogenic pathway
[64]	Carbaryl/naphthalene and chlorpyrifos	Human	Altered semen quality, sperm motility
[65]	BPA	Human	Lower sperm count, abnormal sperm morphology, higher FSH, lower inhibin B level, lower estradiol-to-testosterone ratio
[67]	Dioxin	Human	Higher percentage of oligospermia and abnormal sperm morphology
[10]	Phthalate, Vinclozolin, PBDE	Human	TDS

Table 2.
A summary of the remarkable studies on effects of EDCs on male reproductive systems.

Mixtures of polychlorinated dibenzo-p-dioxins (PCDDs) and dibenzofurans (PCDFs), shortly named 'dioxins', produce adverse health effects reported in several studies. For instance, A study have reported a potential association between chemical dioxins exposure and semen quality. Exposed men have a higher percentage of oligospermia and abnormal sperm morphology [67].

6.2 Testicular cancer, cryptorchidism and hypospadias

Testicular cancer is the most common disorder found in most young men in many countries. A worldwide trend can be observed towards the increasing number of testicular cancers. Exposure to environmental contaminants such as phthalates causes low semen quality, which ultimately may coincide with the development of cryptorchidism, testicular cancer, and hypospadias. The combination of the three aforementioned disorders of the male reproductive system can be termed as "so-called" testicular TDS. Experimental and epidemiological evidence has demonstrated that TDS is an outcome of interference during embryonal physiological programming and gonadal development in fetal life [68, 69]. EDCs such as phthalates, vinclozolin, polybrominated diphenyl ethers (PBDE), and acetaminophen have shown a significant etiopathogenetic role towards the onset of TDS [10]. Despite all these studies, the exact contribution and mechanism behind pesticide and EDC exposure towards testicular cancer development have not been elucidated to date. However, genetic and environmental factors have been documented for the reduced sperm count and disease formation (**Table 2**) [70].

7. Effect of EDCs on fetal and neonatal stages

Although adult exposure towards EDCs is an essential factor, the duration of EDCs exposure in fetus and neonate is also of primary concern. It plays a crucial factor in determining its fate. For instance, Due to early EDCs exposure, development is compromised because EDCs at the neonatal stage are extremely sensitive and affect the same brain regions, circuits, hormone-sensitive pathways, and receptors like the endogenous hormones. Such effects have been reported for several EDCs across various species and have profound detrimental consequences in developing organisms compared to adults [71, 72]. The extreme sensitivity of developing fetus and neonate has been described briefly in a chapter titled "The Fragile Fetus" by Howard Bern [73]. All those protective mechanisms present in adults like DNA Repair Mechanism, detoxifying enzymes, liver metabolism, competent immune system, and the blood–brain barrier are not fully developed or functional during the fetus or neonatal stage. Even the metabolic rate of developing organisms is much higher than adults, which may be the cause of increased toxicity due to environmental contaminants exposures. Numerous reports have documented that developmental exposure to EDCs can lead to various adverse effects in adults and sometimes cause tumors in endocrine tissues and adverse reproductive consequences in males and females [74]. Pieces of evidence have stated that exposure to environmental triggers such as EDCs during critical stages in fetal sex differentiation and development in utero disrupts reproductive organ differentiation and sometimes leading to intersex variation (IV) conditions. IV can be defined as a morphological and physiological anomaly where an individual is born with a congenital condition such as ambiguous genitalia/ hermaphrodite or pseudohermaphroditism etc. [75]. The most evident case for endocrine disruption in utero that may lead to the onset of adult disease in the newborn is prenatal exposure to DES. Between 1958 and 1976, doctors prescribed synthetic estrogen to pregnant women to prevent miscarriages and premature delivery. It was almost a 4-6million pregnancies that were treated with DES in the US alone. In 1971, DES was linked with a rare gynecologic neoplasm in female offspring of DES-exposed pregnancies [76]. Subsequent studies have documented the link between maternal treatment with DES and cervicovaginal cancer in DES-exposed daughters, usually in their late teens or early 20s. This was the first evidence of transplacental carcinogenesis in humans [51]. Additionally, the offspring of DES-exposed mothers also had functional and anatomical abnormalities of the uterus and fallopian tubes.

8. Effect of EDCs on epigenetic regulations

The epigenetic modifications can be defined as "heritable and reversible chemical modifications of chromatin, resulting in an adjustment of its activity without a change in the underlying DNA sequence [77]. Notably, epigenetic effects are mediated by those transcription factors that enhance or repress any specific genes' transcription. The well-studied epigenetic modifications include DNA methylation at the cytosine base, post-translational modification of histone proteins (histone acetylation and deacetylation), and non-coding RNAs. Post-translational modification of histone protein at specific amino acids, for instance, lysine, may alter chromatin's structure and function. Generally, acetylation of histone at lysine position results in activation of transcription by relaxing the chromatin structure, while methylation of lysine depending on the position may lead to activation or repression of gene expression. However, deacetylation may lead to transcriptional repression or silencing of the genes. Non-coding RNA is the transcript of gene sequences that do not code for proteins but regulate its expression in a cis or trans manner mainly involved in some unique functions such as genomic imprinting, X-chromosome inactivation, and developmental patterning and differentiation [70].

The most commonly studied epigenetic mechanism is the EDCs effect on the enzymes that regulate epigenetic patterning, especially the DNA methyl transferase (DNMTs). The endocrine disruptor, Vincolozolin, an androgen receptor antagonist, induced increased expression of dnmt mRNA expression in an in-vivo model through an AR-mediated pathway [78]. Studies have reported that DES can activate immediately early genes such as c-myc, c-jun, c-fos, and lactoferrin, which are upregulated during childhood [53]. This activation is possible due to the promoter region's hypomethylation of the lactoferrin gene in the adult uterus [79]; however, no such patterns were observed when an adult was exposed during adulthood at the same interval. Upon prenatal exposure to DES, tet1 mRNA expression was significantly decreased in mouse uterus and the same response found in zebrafish gonads upon BPA exposure [21, 80, 81]. Exposure to EDCs during development could alter the perturbation of the genome's epigenetic patterning and may result in adult-onset disease. The epigenetic changes in the ovary have been reported for the organochlorine pesticide MTX. In a study, MTX exposure from embryonic to postnatal days caused hypermethylation in the ERβ promoter regions by performing DNA methylation analysis using bisulfite sequencing and methylation-specific PCR [82].

9. Conclusion

Research over the last few years exploited the adverse effects of EDCs, which were lesser-known. Some of them were heavily used in the past decade, and some are just enlisted their names on the list of 'emerging pollutants,' and altogether, they are creating an unhealthy world to live on for us as well as for other animals. This chapter summarizes the harmful effects of EDCs exposure on male and female reproductive physiology and also elucidates the possible mechanism of actions. Though numerous articles and reports regarding these EDCs' toxicological effects are available today, still very little is known about their mechanism of action in our body. The poor understanding of their underlying mechanism in hampering one's endocrine system keeps us at bay to fight against it. Be it your morning toothpaste or your hair nourishing shampoo, and you cannot escape from the exposure of EDCs in your daily life. Even processed foods have EDCs in them. Scientists predict that there are many more of this kind of chemical whose effects are yet to be evaluated. Many countries' government bodies are actively monitoring the situations and taking actions accordingly alongside the scientists who are tirelessly working to find out ways to nullify the adverse effects. We can follow the recent resources available in the public domains and choose a healthy way to live to minimize the EDCs exposure. Extra care should be taken in choosing your packaged food materials, cosmetics, plastic made equipment, cooking utensils, fruits, and vegetables. Finally, emphasis should be on the betterment of regulatory systems for introducing new, untested chemicals alongside the continuous use of chemicals already proved for being EDCs. Utmost care should be taken for pregnant women and infants, who are most vulnerable to EDCs exposure.

Acknowledgements

All authors thank Banaras Hindu University, India for providing necessary resources and support to write the present chapter with the support from University Grant Commission (UGC)-Junior Research Fellowship to PG, AM, and AS. This work received no external funding from any agency.

Conflict of interest

The author declares that there is no conflict of interest.

Author contributions

All authors listed have made a substantial contribution in this chapter. And special thanks to AM for making the required illustrations for this chapter. Thanks to RKS for reviewing the manuscript before the final submission.

Author details

Priya Gupta, Archisman Mahapatra, Anjali Suman and Rahul Kumar Singh*
Molecular Endocrinology and Toxicology Lab (METLab), Department of Zoology, Institute of Science, Banaras Hindu University, Varanasi, India

*Address all correspondence to: rks.rna@gmail.com

References

[1] W. Mnif, A.I.H. Hassine, A. Bouaziz, A. Bartegi, O. Thomas, B. Roig, Effect of endocrine disruptor pesticides: A review, Int. J. Environ. Res. Public Health. 8 (2011) 2265-2303. https://doi.org/10.3390/ijerph8062265.

[2] T.T. Schug, A. Janesick, B. Blumberg, J.J. Heindel, Endocrine disrupting chemicals and disease susceptibility, J. Steroid Biochem. Mol. Biol. 127 (2011) 204-215. https://doi.org/10.1016/j.jsbmb.2011.08.007.

[3] S. De Coster, N. Van Larebeke, Endocrine-disrupting chemicals: Associated disorders and mechanisms of action, J. Environ. Public Health. 2012 (2012). https://doi.org/10.1155/2012/713696.

[4] G.J. Nohynek, C.J. Borgert, D. Dietrich, K.K. Rozman, Endocrine disruption: Fact or urban legend?, Toxicol. Lett. 223 (2013) 295-305. https://doi.org/10.1016/j.toxlet.2013.10.022.

[5] E.R. Kabir, M.S. Rahman, I. Rahman, A review on endocrine disruptors and their possible impacts on human health, Environ. Toxicol. Pharmacol. 40 (2015) 241-258. https://doi.org/10.1016/j.etap.2015.06.009.

[6] R. Kiyama, Y. Wada-Kiyama, Estrogenic endocrine disruptors: Molecular mechanisms of action, Environ. Int. 83 (2015) 11-40. https://doi.org/10.1016/j.envint.2015.05.012.

[7] S. Opinion, Scientific Opinion on the hazard assessment of endocrine disruptors: Scientific criteria for identification of endocrine disruptors and appropriateness of existing test methods for assessing effects mediated by these substances on human health and the env, EFSA J. 11 (2013). https://doi.org/10.2903/j.efsa.2013.3132.

[8] R. Slama, J.P. Bourguignon, B. Demeneix, R. Ivell, G. Panzica, A. Kortenkamp, R.T. Zoeller, Scientific issues relevant to setting regulatory criteria to identify endocrine-disrupting substances in the european union, Environ. Health Perspect. 124 (2016) 1497-1503. https://doi.org/10.1289/EHP217.

[9] B. Yilmaz, H. Terekeci, S. Sandal, F. Kelestimur, Endocrine disrupting chemicals: exposure, effects on human health, mechanism of action, models for testing and strategies for prevention, Rev. Endocr. Metab. Disord. 21 (2020) 127-147. https://doi.org/10.1007/s11154-019-09521-z.

[10] R. Lauretta, A. Sansone, M. Sansone, F. Romanelli, M. Appetecchia, Endocrine disrupting chemicals: Effects on endocrine glands, Front. Endocrinol. (Lausanne). 10 (2019) 1-7. https://doi.org/10.3389/fendo.2019.00178.

[11] C. Monneret, What is an endocrine disruptor?, Comptes Rendus - Biol. 340 (2017) 403-405. https://doi.org/10.1016/j.crvi.2017.07.004.

[12] R. Chaube, S. Mishra, R.K. Singh, In vitro effects of lead nitrate on steroid profiles in the post-vitellogenic ovary of the catfish Heteropneustes fossilis, Toxicol. Vitr. 24 (2010) 1899-1904. https://doi.org/10.1016/j.tiv.2010.07.021.

[13] A. Tokuç, Stockholm Convention (2001) BT - Encyclopedia of Corporate Social Responsibility, in: S.O. Idowu, N. Capaldi, L. Zu, A. Das Gupta (Eds.), Springer Berlin Heidelberg, Berlin, Heidelberg, 2013: pp. 2329-2336. https://doi.org/10.1007/978-3-642-28036-8_15.

[14] UNEP, Stockholm Convention on Persistent Organic Pollutants, (2014). http://www.pops.int/TheConvention/

ThePOPs/TheNewPOPs/tabid/2511/Default.aspx.

[15] O. Yang, H.L. Kim, J.-I. Weon, Y.R. Seo, Endocrine-disrupting Chemicals: Review of Toxicological Mechanisms Using Molecular Pathway Analysis, J. Cancer Prev. 20 (2015) 12-24. https://doi.org/10.15430/jcp.2015.20.1.12.

[16] P. Balaguer, V. Delfosse, M. Grimaldi, W. Bourguet, Structural and functional evidences for the interactions between nuclear hormone receptors and endocrine disruptors at low doses, Comptes Rendus - Biol. 340 (2017) 414-420. https://doi.org/10.1016/j.crvi.2017.08.002.

[17] A.C. Gore, V.A. Chappell, S.E. Fenton, J.A. Flaws, A. Nadal, G.S. Prins, J. Toppari, R.T. Zoeller, EDC-2: The Endocrine Society's Second Scientific Statement on Endocrine-Disrupting Chemicals., Endocr. Rev. 36 (2015) E1–E150. https://doi.org/10.1210/er.2015-1010.

[18] S.P. Bliss, A.M. Navratil, J. Xie, M.S. Roberson, GnRH signaling, the gonadotrope and endocrine control of fertility, Front. Neuroendocrinol. 31 (2010) 322-340. https://doi.org/10.1016/j.yfrne.2010.04.002.

[19] S.A. Sower, M. Freamat, S.I. Kavanaugh, The origins of the vertebrate hypothalamic-pituitary-gonadal (HPG) and hypothalamic-pituitary-thyroid (HPT) endocrine systems: New insights from lampreys, Gen. Comp. Endocrinol. 161 (2009) 20-29. https://doi.org/10.1016/j.ygcen.2008.11.023.

[20] I. Huhtaniemi, A short evolutionary history of FSH-stimulated spermatogenesis, Hormones. 14 (2015) 468-478.

[21] Y. Liu, Y. Zhang, S. Tao, Y. Guan, T. Zhang, Z. Wang, Global DNA methylation in gonads of adult zebrafish Danio rerio under bisphenol A exposure, Ecotoxicol. Environ. Saf. 130 (2016) 124-132. https://doi.org/10.1016/j.ecoenv.2016.04.012.

[22] S.E. Wirbisky, J.L. Freeman, Atrazine exposure and reproductive dysfunction through the Hypothalamus-Pituitary-Gonadal (HPG) axis, Toxics. 3 (2015) 414-450. https://doi.org/10.3390/toxics3040414.

[23] M. Talas, F. Gazárek, J. Stehlíková, H. Fingerová, Serum FSH and LH levels in the normal menstrual cycle, amenorrhea and oligomenorrhea., Endocrinol. Exp. 7 (1973) 80-84.

[24] A.C. Gore, Neuroendocrine targets of endocrine disruptors, Hormones. 9 (2010) 16-27. https://doi.org/10.14310/horm.2002.1249.

[25] S. Hiller-Sturmhöfel, A. Bartke, The endocrine system: an overview., Alcohol Health Res. World. 22 (1998) 153-164.

[26] K. Svechnikov, G. Izzo, L. Landreh, J. Weisser, O. Sder, Endocrine disruptors and leydig cell function, J. Biomed. Biotechnol. 2010 (2010). https://doi.org/10.1155/2010/684504.

[27] E. Laurenzana, G. Balasubramanian, C. Weis, B. Blaydes, R. Newbold, K. Delclos, Effect of nonylphenol on serum testosterone levels and testicular steroidogenic enzyme activity in neonatal, pubertal, and adult rats, Chem. Biol. Interact. 139 (2002) 23-41. https://doi.org/10.1016/S0009-2797(01)00291-5.

[28] P.M.D. Foster, Mode of action: Impaired fetal leydig cell function - Effects on male reproductive development produced by certain phthalate esters, Crit. Rev. Toxicol. 35 (2005) 713-719. https://doi.org/10.1080/10408440591007395.

[29] L. Ye, B. Zhao, G. Hu, Y. Chu, R.S. Ge, Inhibition of human and

rat testicular steroidogenic enzyme activities by bisphenol A, Toxicol. Lett. 207 (2011) 137-142. https://doi.org/10.1016/j.toxlet.2011.09.001.

[30] J.S. Fisher, Environmental anti-androgens and male reproductive health: Focus on phthalates and testicular dysgenesis syndrome, Reproduction. 127 (2004) 305-315. https://doi.org/10.1530/rep.1.00025.

[31] K. Cheshenko, F. Pakdel, H. Segner, O. Kah, R.I.L. Eggen, Interference of endocrine disrupting chemicals with aromatase CYP19 expression or activity, and consequences for reproduction of teleost fish, Gen. Comp. Endocrinol. 155 (2008) 31-62. https://doi.org/10.1016/j.ygcen.2007.03.005.

[32] J.Y. Kim, E.H. Han, H.G. Kim, K.N. Oh, S.K. Kim, K.Y. Lee, H.G. Jeong, Bisphenol A-induced aromatase activation is mediated by cyclooxygenase-2 up-regulation in rat testicular Leydig cells, Toxicol. Lett. 193 (2010) 200-208. https://doi.org/10.1016/j.toxlet.2010.01.011.

[33] G.G.J.M. Kuiper, J.G. Lemmen, B. Carlsson, J.C. Corton, S.H. Safe, P.T. Van Der Saag, B. Van Der Burg, J.Å. Gustafsson, Interaction of estrogenic chemicals and phytoestrogens with estrogen receptor β, Endocrinology. 139 (1998) 4252-4263. https://doi.org/10.1210/endo.139.10.6216.

[34] U. Tiemann, In vivo and in vitro effects of the organochlorine pesticides DDT, TCPM, methoxychlor, and lindane on the female reproductive tract of mammals: A review, Reprod. Toxicol. 25 (2008) 316-326. https://doi.org/10.1016/j.reprotox.2008.03.002.

[35] B. Senthilkumaran, Pesticide- and sex steroid analogue-induced endocrine disruption differentially targets hypothalamo-hypophyseal-gonadal system during gametogenesis in teleosts - A review, Gen. Comp. Endocrinol. 219 (2015). https://doi.org/10.1016/j.ygcen.2015.01.010.

[36] G. Lemaire, W. Mnif, P. Mauvais, P. Balaguer, R. Rahmani, Activation of α- and β-estrogen receptors by persistent pesticides in reporter cell lines, Life Sci. 79 (2006) 1160-1169. https://doi.org/10.1016/j.lfs.2006.03.023.

[37] A. Rajakumar, R. Singh, S. Chakrabarty, R. Murugananthkumar, C. Laldinsangi, Y. Prathibha, C.C. Sudhakumari, A. Dutta-Gupta, B. Senthilkumaran, Endosulfan and flutamide impair testicular development in the juvenile Asian catfish, Clarias batrachus, Aquat. Toxicol. 110-111 (2012) 123-132. https://doi.org/10.1016/j.aquatox.2011.12.018.

[38] W. V. Welshons, K.A. Thayer, B.M. Judy, J.A. Taylor, E.M. Curran, F.S. vom Saal, Large effects from small exposures. I. Mechanisms for endocrine-disrupting chemicals with estrogenic activity, Environ. Health Perspect. 111 (2003) 994-1006. https://doi.org/10.1289/ehp.5494.

[39] W.R. Kelce, C.R. Stone, S.C. Laws, L.E. Gray, J.A. Kemppainen, E.M. Wilson, Persistent DDT metabolite p,p'-DDE is a potent androgen receptor antagonist., Nature. 375 (1995) 581-585. https://doi.org/10.1038/375581a0.

[40] K. Moriyama, T. Tagami, T. Akamizu, T. Usui, M. Saijo, N. Kanamoto, Y. Hataya, A. Shimatsu, H. Kuzuya, K. Nakao, Thyroid hormone action is disrupted by bisphenol A as an antagonist, J. Clin. Endocrinol. Metab. 87 (2002) 5185-5190. https://doi.org/10.1210/jc.2002-020209.

[41] Y.B. Wetherill, N.L. Fisher, A. Staubach, M. Danielsen, R.W. De Vere White, K.E. Knudsen, Xenoestrogen action in prostate cancer: Pleiotropic effects dependent on androgen receptor status, Cancer Res. 65 (2005) 54-65.

[42] J. Peretz, R.K. Gupta, J. Singh, I. Hernández-Ochoa, J.A. Flaws, Bisphenol A impairs follicle growth, inhibits steroidogenesis, and downregulates rate-limiting enzymes in the estradiol biosynthesis pathway, Toxicol. Sci. 119 (2011) 209-217. https://doi.org/10.1093/toxsci/kfq319.

[43] M.C. Rao, a R. Midgley, J.S. Richards, Proliferation of Ovarian Cellular, Cell. 14 (1978) 71-78.

[44] E.M.F. Costa, P.M. Spritzer, A. Hohl, T.A.S.S. Bachega, Effects of endocrine disruptors in the development of the female reproductive tract, Arq. Bras. Endocrinol. Metabol. 58 (2014) 153-161. https://doi.org/10.1590/0004-2730000003031.

[45] C.A. Stratakis, A. Vottero, A. Brodie, L.S. Kirschner, D. Deatkine, Q. Lu, W. Yue, C.S. Mitsiades, A.W. Flor, G.P. Chrousos, The aromatase excess syndrome is associated with feminization of both sexes and autosomal dominant transmission of aberrant p450 aromatase gene transcription, J. Clin. Endocrinol. Metab. 83 (1998) 1348-1357. https://doi.org/10.1210/jc.83.4.1348.

[46] G.D. Braunstein, Aromatase and gynecomastia, Endocr. Relat. Cancer. 6 (1999) 315-324. https://doi.org/10.1677/erc.0.0060315.

[47] C. Brisken, Endocrine disruptors and breast cancer, Chimia (Aarau). 62 (2008) 406-409. https://doi.org/10.2533/chimia.2008.406.

[48] N. Ben-Jonathan, Endocrine Disrupting Chemicals and Breast Cancer: The Saga of Bisphenol A, in: X. Zhang (Ed.), Estrogen Recept. Breast Cancer Celebr. 60th Anniv. Discov. ER, Springer International Publishing, Cham, 2019: pp. 343-377. https://doi.org/10.1007/978-3-319-99350-8_13.

[49] J.R. Palmer, L.A. Wise, E.E. Hatch, R. Troisi, L. Titus-Ernstoff, W. Strohsnitter, R. Kaufman, A.L. Herbst, K.L. Noller, M. Hyer, R.N. Hoover, Prenatal diethylstilbestrol exposure and risk of breast cancer., Cancer Epidemiol. Biomarkers Prev. a Publ. Am. Assoc. Cancer Res. Cosponsored by Am. Soc. Prev. Oncol. 15 (2006) 1509-1514. https://doi.org/10.1158/1055-9965.EPI-06-0109.

[50] L. Lucaccioni, V. Trevisani, L. Marrozzini, N. Bertoncelli, B. Predieri, L. Lugli, A. Berardi, L. Iughetti, Endocrine-Disrupting Chemicals and Their Effects during Female Puberty: A Review of Current Evidence., Int. J. Mol. Sci. 21 (2020). https://doi.org/10.3390/ijms21062078.

[51] J.A. McLachlan, E. Simpson, M. Martin, Endocrine disrupters and female reproductive health., Best Pract. Res. Clin. Endocrinol. Metab. 20 (2006) 63-75. https://doi.org/10.1016/j.beem.2005.09.009.

[52] M. Morgan, A. Deoraj, Q. Felty, D. Roy, Environmental estrogen-like endocrine disrupting chemicals and breast cancer., Mol. Cell. Endocrinol. 457 (2017) 89-102. https://doi.org/10.1016/j.mce.2016.10.003.

[53] N. L.M., Clinical practice. Primary ovarian insufficiency., N. Engl. J. Med. 360 (2009) 606-614.

[54] R.R. Newbold, W.N. Jefferson, E. Padilla-Banks, Prenatal Exposure to Bisphenol A at environmentally relevant doses adversely affects the murine female reproductive tract later in life, Environ. Health Perspect. 117 (2009) 879-885. https://doi.org/10.1289/ehp.0800045.

[55] M. Uzumcu, P.E. Kuhn, J.E. Marano, A.M.E. Armenti, L. Passantino, Early postnatal methoxychlor exposure inhibits folliculogenesis and stimulates anti-Mullerian hormone production

in the rat ovary, J. Endocrinol. 191 (2006) 549-558. https://doi.org/10.1677/joe.1.06592.

[56] A. Kirigaya, H. Kim, S. Hayashi, P. Chambon, H. Watanabe, T. Iguchi, T. Sato, Involvement of estrogen receptor β in the induction of polyovular follicles in mouse ovaries exposed neonatally to diethylstilbestrol, Zoolog. Sci. 26 (2009) 704-712. https://doi.org/10.2108/zsj.26.704.

[57] H.R. Chao, S.L. Wang, L.Y. Lin, W.J. Lee, O. Päpke, Placental transfer of polychlorinated dibenzo-p-dioxins, dibenzofurans, and biphenyls in Taiwanese mothers in relation to menstrual cycle characteristics, Food Chem. Toxicol. 45 (2007) 259-265. https://doi.org/10.1016/j.fct.2006.07.032.

[58] Y. Nikaido, K. Yoshizawa, N. Danbara, M. Tsujita-Kyutoku, T. Yuri, N. Uehara, A. Tsubura, Effects of maternal xenoestrogen exposure on development of the reproductive tract and mammary gland in female CD-1 mouse offspring, Reprod. Toxicol. 18 (2004) 803-811. https://doi.org/10.1016/j.reprotox.2004.05.002.

[59] B.S. Rubin, J.R. Lenkowski, C.M. Schaeberle, L.N. Vandenberg, P.M. Ronsheim, A.M. Soto, Evidence of altered brain sexual differentiation in mice exposed perinatally to low, environmentally relevant levels of bisphenol A, Endocrinology. 147 (2006) 3681-3691. https://doi.org/10.1210/en.2006-0189.

[60] P. Alonso-Magdalena, S. Morimoto, C. Ripoll, E. Fuentes, A. Nadal, The estrogenic effect of bisphenol a disrupts pancreatic β-cell function in vivo and induces insulin resistance, Environ. Health Perspect. 114 (2006) 106-112. https://doi.org/10.1289/ehp.8451.

[61] M. Axelstad, U. Hass, M. Scholze, S. Christiansen, A. Kortenkamp, J. Boberg, EDC IMPACT: Reduced sperm counts in rats exposed to human relevant mixtures of endocrine disrupters, Endocr. Connect. 7 (2018) 139-148. https://doi.org/10.1530/EC-17-0307.

[62] S. Rehman, Z. Usman, S. Rehman, M. AlDraihem, N. Rehman, I. Rehman, G. Ahmad, Endocrine disrupting chemicals and impact on male reproductive health, Transl. Androl. Urol. 7 (2018) 490-503. https://doi.org/10.21037/tau.2018.05.17.

[63] C. Quan, C. Wang, P. Duan, W. Huang, W. Chen, S. Tang, K. Yang, Bisphenol a induces autophagy and apoptosis concurrently involving the Akt/mTOR pathway in testes of pubertal SD rats., Environ. Toxicol. 32 (2017) 1977-1989. https://doi.org/10.1002/tox.22339.

[64] J.D. Meeker, L. Ryan, D.B. Barr, R.F. Herrick, D.H. Bennett, R. Bravo, R. Hauser, The relationship of urinary metabolites of carbaryl/naphthalene and chlorpyrifos with human semen quality, Environ. Health Perspect. 112 (2004) 1665-1670. https://doi.org/10.1289/ehp.7234.

[65] J.D. Meeker, S. Ehrlich, T.L. Toth, D.L. Wright, A.M. Calafat, A.T. Trisini, X. Ye, R. Hauser, Semen quality and sperm DNA damage in relation to urinary bisphenol A among men from an infertility clinic, Reprod. Toxicol. 30 (2010) 532-539. https://doi.org/10.1016/j.reprotox.2010.07.005.

[66] J. Mendiola, N. Jørgensen, A.M. Andersson, A.M. Calafat, X. Ye, J.B. Redmon, E.Z. Drobnis, C. Wang, A. Sparks, S.W. Thurston, F. Liu, S.H. Swan, Are environmental levels of bisphenol A associated with reproductive function in fertile men?, Environ. Health Perspect. 118 (2010) 1286-1291. https://doi.org/10.1289/ehp.1002037.

[67] A.C. Faure, J.F. Viel, A. Bailly, O. Blagosklonov, C. Amiot, C. Roux,

Evolution of sperm quality in men living in the vicinity of a municipal solid waste incinerator possibly correlated with decreasing dioxins emission levels, Andrologia. 46 (2014) 744-752. https://doi.org/10.1111/and.12143.

[68] N.E. Skakkebaek, E. Rajpert-De Meyts, K.M. Main, Testicular dysgenesis syndrome: an increasingly common developmental disorder with environmental aspects., Hum. Reprod. 16 (2001) 972-978. https://doi.org/10.1093/humrep/16.5.972.

[69] H.E. Virtanen, M. Kaleva, A.M. Haavisto, I.M. Schmidt, M. Chellakooty, K.M. Main, N.E. Skakkebaek, J. Toppari, The birth rate of hypospadias in the Turku area in Finland., APMIS. 109 (2001) 96-100. https://doi.org/10.1034/j.1600-0463.2001.d01-109.x.

[70] S. Sifakis, V.P. Androutsopoulos, A.M. Tsatsakis, D.A. Spandidos, Human exposure to endocrine disrupting chemicals: effects on the male and female reproductive systems., Environ. Toxicol. Pharmacol. 51 (2017) 56-70. https://doi.org/10.1016/j.etap.2017.02.024.

[71] A.C. Gore, Developmental programming and endocrine disruptor effects on reproductive neuroendocrine systems, Front. Neuroendocrinol. 29 (2008) 358-374. https://doi.org/10.1016/j.yfrne.2008.02.002.

[72] D.J.P. Barker, The developmental origins of adult disease., Eur. J. Epidemiol. 18 (2003) 733-736. https://doi.org/10.1023/a:1025388901248.

[73] B. HA, Chemically-Induced Alterations in Sexual and Functional Development: The Wildlife/Human Connection., in: C.C. Colborn T. (Ed.), The Fragile Fetus, Princeton Scientific Publishing Co Inc.; Princeton, 1992: pp. 9-15.

[74] R.R. Newbold, E. Padilla-Banks, R.J. Snyder, T.M. Phillips, W.N. Jefferson, Developmental exposure to endocrine disruptors and the obesity epidemic, Reprod. Toxicol. 23 (2007) 290-296. https://doi.org/10.1016/j.reprotox.2006.12.010.

[75] A.L. Rich, L.M. Phipps, S. Tiwari, H. Rudraraju, P.O. Dokpesi, The Increasing Prevalence in Intersex Variation from Toxicological Dysregulation in Fetal Reproductive Tissue Differentiation and Development by Endocrine-Disrupting Chemicals, Environ. Health Insights. 10 (2016) EHI.S39825. https://doi.org/10.4137/EHI.S39825.

[76] A.L. Herbst, H. Ulfelder, D.C. Poskanzer, Adenocarcinoma of the vagina. Association of maternal stilbestrol therapy with tumor appearance in young women., N. Engl. J. Med. 284 (1971) 878-881. https://doi.org/10.1056/NEJM197104222841604.

[77] S. Santangeli, F. Maradonna, I. Olivotto, C.C. Piccinetti, G. Gioacchini, O. Carnevali, Effects of BPA on female reproductive function: The involvement of epigenetic mechanism, Gen. Comp. Endocrinol. 245 (2017) 122-126. https://doi.org/10.1016/j.ygcen.2016.08.010.

[78] P.A. Cowin, E. Gold, J. Aleksova, M.K. O'Bryan, P.M.D. Foster, H.S. Scott, G.P. Risbridger, Vinclozolin exposure in utero induces postpubertal prostatitis and reduces sperm production via a reversible hormone-regulated mechanism, Endocrinology. 151 (2010) 783-792. https://doi.org/10.1210/en.2009-0982.

[79] S. Li, K.A. Washburn, R. Moore, T. Uno, C. Teng, R.R. Newbold, J.A. McLachlan, M. Negishi, Developmental exposure to diethylstilbestrol elicits demethylation of estrogen-responsive lactoferrin gene in mouse uterus, Cancer Res. 57 (1997) 4356-4359.

[80] W.N. Jefferson, D.M. Chevalier, J.Y. Phelps, A.M. Cantor, E. Padilla-Banks, R.R. Newbold, T.K. Archer, H. Karimi Kinyamu, C.J. Williams, Persistently altered epigenetic marks in the mouse uterus after neonatal estrogen exposure, Mol. Endocrinol. 27 (2013) 1666-1677. https://doi.org/10.1210/me.2013-1211.

[81] A. Alavian-Ghavanini, J. Rüegg, Understanding Epigenetic Effects of Endocrine Disrupting Chemicals: From Mechanisms to Novel Test Methods, Basic Clin. Pharmacol. Toxicol. 122 (2018) 38-45. https://doi.org/10.1111/bcpt.12878.

[82] A.M. Zama, M. Uzumcu, Fetal and neonatal exposure to the endocrine disruptor methoxychlor causes epigenetic alterations in adult ovarian genes, Endocrinology. 150 (2009) 4681-4691. https://doi.org/10.1210/en.2009-0499.

Chapter 3

Environmental Obesogens and Human Health

Archisman Mahapatra, Priya Gupta, Anjali Suman and Rahul Kumar Singh

Abstract

Obesity is an alarming public health concern that contributes to a substantially increased risk of multiple chronic disorders, including diabetes. As per WHO data, in 2016, almost 39% adult population of the world is overweight, 13% of them were obese. There is prominent evidence on the involvement of environmental endocrine-disrupting chemicals, termed obesogens, in the prevalence of this growing worldwide pandemic, obesity. The exaggerated effect of obesogens on endocrine disruption, lipid metabolism and homeostasis, adipocyte functioning, impaired thermogenesis, inflammation, epigenetics, and overall human health will be covered in this chapter. This chapter will discuss the environmental obesogen hypothesis, the epidemiological and experimental evidence of obesogens, its chemical characteristics, and possible mechanism of actions. It will also focus on some recent indications of obesogens and their correlation in COVID-19 disease pathogenesis. This chapter will try to conclude with strategies for identifying the underlying mechanisms of obesogens within model systems and the human body, including future directions.

Keywords: endocrine disrupting chemicals, obesogens, obesity, gut microbiota, peroxisome proliferator-activated receptor γ, lipid metabolism, energy homeostasis

1. Introduction

1.1 Endocrine-disrupting chemicals

As defined by the US Environmental Protection Agency (EPA) [1], an endocrine-disrupting chemical (EDCs) is "an exogenous agent that interferes with synthesis, secretion, transport, metabolism, binding action, or elimination of natural blood-borne hormones that are present in the body and are responsible for homeostasis, reproduction, and developmental process." Diamanti-Kandarakis et al. [2] among thousands of human-made chemicals, almost 1000 chemicals may have endocrine-disrupting properties [3]. Initially, it was thought that EDCs deploy their actions mainly through various nuclear hormone receptors like estrogen receptors (ERs), progesterone receptors (PRs), androgen receptors (ARs) and thyroid receptors. However, as research progressed on EDCs and their mechanism of actions, it is now known that they can also act on non-nuclear receptors, nonsteroid receptors, orphan receptors and other enzymatic pathways related to metabolism, cancer and other physiological processes [2].

As the compounds classified under EDCs are from dispersed heterogeneous sources, they can be divided into two major classes, synthetic and natural. Synthetic EDCs include industrial solvents and their byproducts [dioxins, polychlorinated biphenyls (PCBs), polybrominated biphenyls (PBBs), alkylphenols etc.], agricultural pesticides [methoxychlor (MTX), chlorpyrifos, dichlorodiphenyltrichloroethane (DDT)], fungicides, herbicides, insecticides, plasticizers [phthalates, bisphenol A (BPA)] and pharmaceuticals [diethylstilbestrol (DES)] whereas, phytoestrogens (genistein, coumestrol etc.) are grouped under natural sources of EDCs. Humans are exposed to the broad range of EDCs mainly through the dietary intake (fish, meat, dairy and poultry products) and to some extent by inhalation and dermal uptake [2, 4]. Mostly EDCs are highly lipophilic, and they tend to get accumulated in the adipose tissues [5, 6]. They can accumulate in human and other large mammals' fatty tissues through biomagnification and bioaccumulation as they are the top predators in the food chain [7]. Due to their long half-life, they remain stored in the adipose tissues for years. Persistent Organic Pollutants (POPs) are the best example of long term accumulations in human tissues [8]. However, plasticizers like BPA have a very short estimated half-life of about four hours. Instead of bioaccumulation, they generally get excreted via urine [9]. Still, BPA has a very adverse effect on the human endocrine system due to their continuous exposure throughout the days [10].

Among the vast range of chemicals under EDCs, some are referred to as "obesogens" as they promote or induce weight gain in individuals by altering endocrine pathways involved in metabolism, energy homeostasis and appetite. The phthalates, perfluorinated compounds, BPA, dioxins, and some pesticides showed obesogenic potentials [11, 12]. Though their mechanism of action is not very well understood, some report indicated that these chemicals might act through Peroxisome proliferator-activated receptor gamma γ (PPAR-γ), a ligand-activated transcription factor, has a role in various cellular functions as well as glucose homeostasis, lipid metabolism, and prevention of oxidative stress [13, 14]. Some suggest they may act via the thyroid axis, as the thyroid hormone is a crucial regulator of metabolism [15, 16]. Hence, this field is relatively new and emerging in EDC's research and needs further studies.

2. Environmental obesogen hypothesis

The prevalence of obesity and associated diseases like type 2 diabetes, cardiovascular diseases, metabolic syndromes and cancers are progressively increasing at an alarming rate in recent years. Globally the cases of obesity have nearly tripled since 1975. As per a WHO report, in 2016, 13% of adults aged 18 or more are obese worldwide. A more recent report stated that approximately thirty-eight million children (under five years) are obese. In simple language, obesity can be defined as an "abnormal or excessive fat accumulation that may impair health" [17]. The measure of obesity is generally done by body mass index (BMI), defined as a person's weight in kilograms divided by the square of his/her height in meters (kg/m^2). A BMI of 30 or greater falls within the obese range; the limit changes to 25 or more in Asian populations [18, 19]. It is a widely accepted fact that the primary cause of obesity is the imbalance between calory intake and energy expenditure. However, obesity is a complex disease caused mainly by endocrine disruption, which also involves interaction between genetic and environmental factors.

The Obesogen Hypothesis suggests that environmental chemicals, characterized as "obesogens," induce obesity by enhancing the engagement, differentiation and size of adipocytes, by altering metabolic setpoints or modifying the hormonal control of appetite and satiety [20]. Many EDCs are obesogens in nature and found abundantly in our environment, which may induce adipogenesis and lipid accumulation in the tissues. About 50 of such compounds have been identified to date [20]. Various mechanisms of action of the obesogens are discussed later in this chapter.

3. Chemical characteristics of obesogens

Obesogens have peculiar characteristics which make them potential to interfere with various endocrine and metabolic pathways. They are believed to be xenohormones as they imitate or partially resemble natural hormones and have unwanted physiological effects. They can bind to endocrine receptors present on the cell membrane, cytosol, or nucleus, thereby altering their natural functions [21]. Along with the structural similarities with native hormones, their ability to do this also relies on its lipophilicity and small molecular weight. Partition coefficient, half-life and molecular weight are the three main components of xenohormones. A partition coefficient (P) is "the ratio of the concentration of a substance in one medium or phase (C1) to the concentration in a second phase (C2) when the two concentrations are at equilibrium; that is, partition coefficient = (C1/C2)equal." [22]. This is how the distribution efficiency of a chemical is measured between two mediums. Here in obesogen's case, it is between the tissue and blood. A compound's octanol–water partition coefficient expresses that (K_{OW}), referred to the ratio of a chemical's concentration in the octanol phase to its concentration in the aqueous phase of a two-phase octanol/water system [23]. It is an essential measure of its lipophilicity of a chemical. The bioaccumulation and toxicity of a chemical largely depend upon

Source	Obesogens	Chemical characteristics		
		Log K_{OW}	Biological Half-life	Mol. weight
Industrial	BPA	3.32	21.3 +/− 7.4 h [26]	228.29 g/mol
	Bisphenol S (BPS)	1.65	6.8 ± 0.7 h [27]	250.27 g/mol
	BDE-47	6.76 [28]	664 days [29]	485.79 g/mol
	3,3′,4,4′-Tetrachlorobiphenyl (PCB-77)	6.72	1.2 Months [30]	292 g/mol
	bis(2-ethylhexyl) phthalate (DEHP)	7.6	12 hours [31]	390.6 g/mol
	Dioxin	6.8	5.8 years [32]	322 g/mol
	Perfluorooctanoic acid	4.81	12.6 days	414.07 g/mol
Pesticides/ insecticides	Dichlorodiphenyl-trichloroethane (DDT)	6.91	7 years [33]	354.5 g/mol
	Tributyltin (TBT)	3.1–4.1 [34]	23–30 days [35]	290.1 g/mol
	Atrazine	2.61	10.8–11.2 hours [36]	215.68 g/mol
Pharmaceuticals	Diethylstilbestrol (DES)	5.07	2–3 days [37]	268.3 g/mol
	Nicotine	1.17	2 h [38]	162.23 g/mol

Note: All values are acquired from the PubChem database otherwise mentioned.

Table 1.
Chemical characteristics of some obesogens.

K_{OW}. As being organic, obesogens are naturally lipophilic compound, which means they have a higher K_{OW} value. More the value of the K_{OW} of a compound, the more will be its tendency to accumulate in the adipose tissues [24].

Now, coming to the half-life, the biological half-life of a chemical is the time it takes to break down or eliminate half of the chemical's quantity from the body. In the body, a longer biological half-life implies longer endurance. Ideally, obesogens have longer biological half-lives means a short exposure can have life-long consequences [25]. The last of the three properties, molecular weight, refers to the size of a compound molecule. Small molecules can diffuse more readily through adipocytes. However, many large molecules having high molecular weight can give rise to smaller metabolites which may have a similar effect to obesogens [24]. The bioaccumulation and the binding affinity for the receptors largely depend upon these three criteria. Many obesogens perfectly fit into these criteria. Moreover, some of them are also resistant to degradation [e.g. 2,2′,4,4′-tetrabromodiphenyl ether (BDE-47)] [21]. A summary of some well-known obesogens with their characteristics is listed in **Table 1**.

4. Mechanisms of action of obesogens

Though the mechanism of obesogens' actions in inducing obesity is not very clear, some studies suggest few mechanisms by which obesogen could act. This disruption of lipid homeostasis by obesogen may involve several mechanisms, some of which are as follows (**Figure 1**):

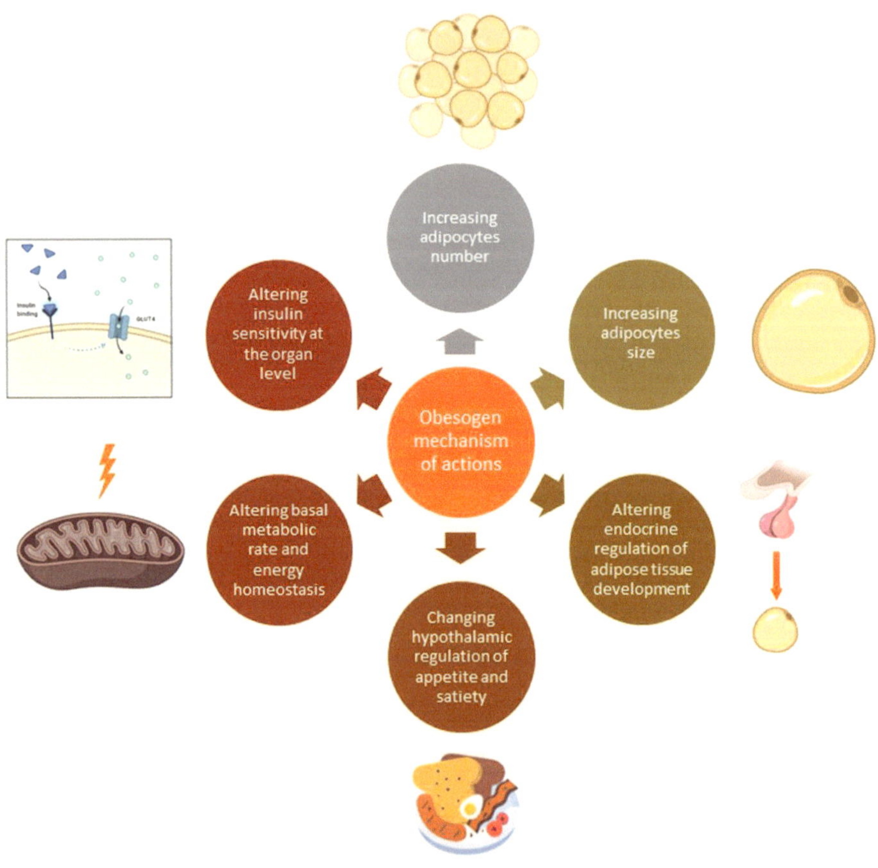

Figure 1.
Mechanisms of obesogen actions.

1. increasing the adipocytes number,

2. increasing the size of the adipocytes,

3. altering endocrine regulation of adipose tissue development,

4. changing hypothalamic regulation of appetite and satiety

5. altering basal metabolic rate and energy homeostasis

6. altering insulin sensitivity at the organ level

4.1 PPARγ-RXR mediated

Obesogens generally disturb the endocrine system by interfering with PPARγ and other hormone receptors like estrogen receptor, androgen receptors and glucocorticoid receptors. PPARγ is one of the primary regulators of adipogenesis. It is highly expressed in adipose tissues and induce differentiation of adipocytes by promoting lipogenic enzymes. Along with adipogenesis, it activates genes involved in maintaining energy balance. Upon activation, PPARγ forms a heterodimer complex with nuclear receptor 9-cis retinoic acid receptor (RXR) an act as promoters for the genes required for storage of fatty acid and repression of lipolysis. That is why this PPARγ:RXR heterodimer is called the "master regulator of adipogenesis" [39]. Obesogen tributyltin (TBT) acts as a ligand and show high binding affinity with PPARγ and nuclear receptor RXR. By activating PPARγ and RXR, it might promote adipogenesis and lipid dysbiosis [40, 41]. Obesogens like spirodiclofen and quinoxyfen activate PPARγ while others like fludioxonil activate RXR [13]. Phthalates are also known activators of PPARγ, as they are shown to promote 3 T3-L1 cells to adipocytes differentiation [42]. Obesogen can increase the amount of adipose tissue by increasing the size as well as numbers of adipocytes. They can induce the Mesenchymal Stem Cells (MSCs) to differentiate into preadipocytes and adipocytes [43]. In vitro assays show numerous compounds with obesogenic properties can induce the Mesenchymal Stem Cells (MSCs) to differentiate into preadipocytes and adipocytes via PPARγ dependent pathways. TBT exposure to 3 T3-L1 preadipocytes induces them to differentiate into white adipose tissues (WAT) [44]. Bisphenol A (BPA), combined with insulin, can accelerate the conversion of 3 T3-L1 fibroblasts to adipocytes [45]. Even prenatal exposure to TBT in mouse shows preferential differentiation of MSCs towards the adipose lineage [43] (**Figure 2**).

From the studies available so far, it is evident that any ligand which can bind to PPARγ can induce adipogenesis and can be called obesogens. However, as human adipose tissue stores many of them, they can have a more significant cumulative effect. These additive effects are not well studied yet.

4.2 Other receptor-mediated

Obesogens are reported to act via other hormone receptors like estrogen receptor, androgen receptors and glucocorticoid receptors. Many studies have reported that they act via the nuclear hormone receptor-mediated pathways. Molecular cross talks with other signaling pathways have also been reported. Steroid hormones have an essential role in lipid storage and disposition of body fat. Estrogen based hormone replacement therapy is prescribed to women at their menopause to remodel their adipose depot. Foetal or neonatal exposure to phytoestrogens may induce

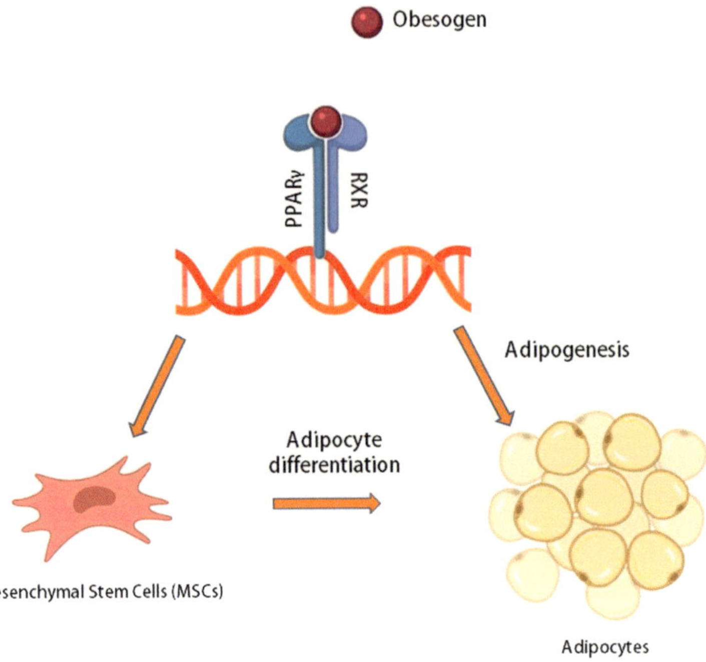

Figure 2.
PPARγ-RXR mediated action of obesogens.

obesity in later stages of life. Well-known phytoestrogen genistein, commonly found in soy-based foods, affects adipose tissue deposition in a dose-dependent and gender-specific manner [46].

Neonatal exposure of DES to female mice led to weight gain in adulthood. However, this effect can be sex-biased. While some EDCs may act directly via cellular steroid receptors by inducing estrogen synthesis, other EDCs may act indirectly. It is established that adipose tissue is a site of estrogen synthesis. The adipocyte cytoplasm contains the enzyme cytochrome P450 aromatase, which plays a vital role in converting estrogen from androgen. It is now reported that several EDCs can impair intracellular aromatase activity [47]. This action may raise intracellular estrogen levels in adipocytes and lead to obesity irrespective of the sexes [48]. It is reported that TBT can directly reduce the activity of the aromatase enzyme in adipose tissue at high doses, leading to reduced estradiol levels and down-regulation of the ER target genes. TBT also has an inhibitory effect on 11β-hydroxysteroid dehydrogenase 2, which leads to reduced inactivation of cortisol. It is believed that increased glucocorticoid levels could influence adipocyte differentiation and regulation of metabolism [40].

Some obesogens, especially the persistent organic pollutants (POPs), act via the ligand-activated transcription factor aryl hydrocarbon receptor (AhR). AhR activates xenobiotic-metabolizing enzyme cytochrome P450s. They can promote adipogenesis indirectly by changing PPARγ expression.

4.3 Other mechanisms

In some recent studies, researchers found that they are not linked to activation of any nuclear hormone receptors; instead, they followed some novel mechanisms, which make their mechanism of action more complex. Those include epigenetic modifications, impairment of thermogenesis and dysbiosis in gut microbiota. Some of these mechanisms will be discussed in the following sections. Some recent studies correlated COVID-19 pandemic to the obesogenic exposures, that is also being discussed in this chapter.

4.3.1 Epigenetic modifications

Epigenetics is defined as the study of heritable changes in phenotype resulting from environmentally influenced modifications of genome. Epigenetic modification can alter gene expression during development and cellular differentiation in response to environmental factors such as chemical contaminants. These modifications include DNA methylation at cytosine residues of 5′ to guanine sites (CpG sites), chemically modifying histone proteins and noncoding RNAs interference [49]. DNA methylation was considered a key mechanism responsible for adult diseases with developmental origins [50]. DNA methylation changes are responsible for the transgenerational effects of exogenous exposed individuals to chemicals and nutrition deficits [51]. For instance, the obesogen pesticide TBT induced changes in DNA methylation and histone modification invitro. Various reports have documented the environmental chemicals, including obesogens, led to an epigenetic modification in vivo and obesogen phenotype even in unexposed generations. TBT exposure in 3 T3-L1 mice preadipocytes invitro resulted in increased adipocyte differentiation along with decreased DNA methylation levels. Increased differentiation level towards the adipogenic lineage was observed in adipose-derived stromal cells (ADSCs) isolated from TBT exposed mice perinatally but at the cost of decreased osteogenesis. ADSCs exposed to TBT were associated with increased adipogenesis marker genes, such as PPARγ target gene Fapb4, where methylation level decreased in the promoter region. However, PPARγ mRNA levels were increased, but DNA methylation at its promoter region had no effects [43]. A possible reason for this lack of epigenetic regulation might be that EDC exposure during differentiation process causes DNA histone demethylation. Ultimately, PPARγ, which is under the control of H3K27me3, causes the gene to be promptly up-regulated. Importantly, prenatal exposure to TBT has been recently shown to cause the transgenerational inheritance of adiposity. It remains to be determined whether these transgenerational effects are related to permanent changes in DNA methylation profiles or other epigenetic processes.

4.3.2 Impairment of thermogenesis

Recent advances found in understanding adipocyte function was the presence of thermogenic brown adipose tissue (BAT) in adult human beings in a dispersed manner, not as found in concentrated discrete depots in human infants. Another discovery of white adipose tissue can also be induced to produce thermogenic fat called beige or brite fat. Increased mitochondria production is responsible for differentiation of both bona fide brown adipocytes and beiging of white adipocytes. This thermogenesis relies on the capacity to dissipate energy in the form of heat through uncoupling of cellular oxidative phosphorylation and ATP synthesis via Uncoupling protein 1 (UCP1) or sometimes through shivering. Some of the evidence has documented how some obesogens impede the production and function of thermogenic adipocytes. For instance, perinatal exposures to DDT in mice have long term-effects on thermogenesis regulation in their female offspring. When female offspring reached up to 6 months of age, they showed reduced energy expenditure & ultimately decreased thermogenesis capacity. However, no change in their physical activity was observed. Thermogenesis impairment was due to the decreased expression of PPAR-γ co-activator 1α (Ppargc1a), a master regulator for thermogenesis related genes and type 2 iodothyronine deiodinase (DiO2) (the enzyme that catalyzes thyroid hormone T4 to convert into T3 which stimulates BAT thermogenesis) [52]. Secondly, Shoucri and his colleagues [49] found that TBT or rexinoids have inhibited adipocytes' production. Other EDCs increase thermogenesis by changing mRNA and protein levels of UCP-1. Adult mice exposed to PFOA and PFOS through diet (containing 0.02% w/w) for ten days exhibited BAT mitochondria activation for increased oxidative capacity and protein levels of UCP-1, resulting in decreased depots size of adipose tissue. PFOA exposure (80–40 μM) during in-vitro experiments activates UCP1 similarly as fatty acids. These examples indicate how obesogens influence obesity by impairing thermogenesis during the in-vitro and in vivo study. This intriguing area of obesogen epidemic and their mechanism remains to be elucidated. Through their Horizon 2020 programme, the European Union has funded several grants to establish new assays to assess EDCs effects on metabolic-end points and identify those chemicals that affect thermogenesis [53].

4.3.3 Gut microbiota dysbiosis

The gut microbiome is defined as "the totality of microorganisms, bacteria, viruses, protozoa, and fungi, and their collective genetic material present in the gastrointestinal tract" by molecular biologist Joshua Lederberg. Obesogen exposure could lead to obesity by altering the gut microbiome, a relatively novel mechanism which leads to obesity. It is well understood that obesity is correlated with gut microbiome composition [54]. Some experimental data shows that the transplant of gut microbe from obese mice can induce obesity in lean mice [55]. Conversely, the gut microbiome transplant from lean donors improved the metabolic disorder condition in obese mice [56]. It is evident from several experimental data that many obesogens induce the gut microbiome dysbiosis in zebrafish [57], mice [58] and human [59]. In mice, gut microbial dysbiosis was associated with increased fat accumulation or impaired lipid metabolism after exposure to triphenyl phosphate. Tributyltin exposure induces gut microbiome dysbiosis with increased body weight gain and dyslipidemia in mice [58]. Though, it is not yet apparent whether this metabolic disruption is a result of the gut microbiota dysbiosis or not.

Additionally, some microbial metabolites have also been reported as AhR agonists and antagonists [60, 61], as we are already aware that activating AhR inhibits adipogenesis. In contrast, inhibition of the activity leads to obesity and fatty liver disease. Two basic dietary emulsifiers, carboxymethylcellulose and P-80, were reported to initiate intestinal inflammation and gut microbiota dysbiosis, which led to metabolic disorder and increased body weight in mice [62]. These pieces of evidence suggest that inducing obesity via gut microbiota dysbiosis is possibly a potent mechanism for the obesogens to follow. However, to get more clues, this field needs to be studied further extensively.

4.3.4 Obesogens and COVID-19

The current outbreak of novel coronavirus has emerged as a worldwide pandemic in the past year, which is related to the Severe Acute Respiratory Syndrome Coronavirus (SARS-CoV) in 2003 and the Middle East Respiratory Syndrome Coronavirus (MERS-CoV) in 2012 [63]. Interestingly, a study in 2003 found a positive correlation between air pollution and extreme SARS in the Chinese population. Patients with SARS from regions with a high air pollution index (API) were twice as likely as those from regions with low APIs to die from SARS [64]. A finding based on US population found that long-term exposure to air pollution resulted in a 6% rise in cardiopulmonary mortality risk. Some of these pollutants are potent obesogenic [65].

Human studies have even shown nitrogen dioxide (NO2), one of the components of air pollution, is correlated with higher fasting serum lipids among obese individuals, indicating that obesity can worsen the effects of air pollution [66]. Animal studies have also shown that air pollution particles' sensitivity early in life will contribute to increased visceral obesity, insulin tolerance, and inflammation, signaling NO2's function as an endocrine disruptor [67]. Since COVID-19 is similar to SARS in causing respiratory disease, exposure to NO2 can increase the mortality rate of patients with COVID-19. However, future studies are needed to validate this relationship.

5. Transgenerational effects

One of the most intriguing results in EDCs field came when a series of reports were published by Skinner and colleagues showing EDCs, including DDT and MTX, induce transgenerational obesogenic effects. During F1 generation, prenatally exposed individuals with anti-androgenic fungicide vinclozolin or estrogenic pesticide MTX were associated with disease in various organs in their F4 generation [68]. Similarly, when pregnant mice (FO generation) were exposed to environmentally relevant doses (nM) of TBT through drinking water, then effects on obesity were observed in F1-F3 descendants of exposed animals [69]. Notably, in a similar experiment, the pharmacological obesogen, Rosiglitazone, which can activate PPARγ, could not produce the same transgenerational obesity effects suggesting that different pathways in addition to PPARγ were required to generate transgenerational phenotype [69].

In addition to TBT effects on obesity, Skinner lab has shown several environmental chemicals such as plasticizer (BPA, DEHP, DBP) [70], pesticides MTX [71], a mixed hydrocarbon mixture (jet fuel JP-8) [72] and the widely used pesticide DDT [73], induced transgenerational obesity in a rat model as observed in F3/F4 offspring of ancestral prenatal or perinatal obesogen exposed-FO individuals [71–73]. Although molecular mechanisms underlying transgenerational inheritance of obesity are currently controversial, researchers belonging to the EDC field believe that these obesogen effects are inherited in an epigenetic manner. This point has got stronger resistance in the genetics sphere [74].

6. Epidemiological evidence of obesogens

6.1 Human cohort studies

Epidemiological studies are of considerable significance for the association of disease effects with exposure to obesogens. Few cohort-based studies are available to date on the effect of obesogens in human populations. Since a considerable amount of evidence indicate that prenatal exposures predispose patients to obesity, epidemiological research concentrates on obesogenic measurements throughout pregnancy. Increase in child adiposity in multiple birth cohorts was associated with prenatal exposure to PFAS. At the same time, sexual dimorphism was sometimes linked with it [75–79]. A metapopulation analysis, including ten cohorts, suggests a 25% and 0.1 unit increase in weight and BMI, respectively, per ng/ml of PFOA concentration in maternal blood [80].

A research found that rising concentrations of maternal urinary phthalate during gestation doubled the risk of the offspring becoming overweight or obese

[81]. Cohort research on the impact of prenatal BPA exposure has also been correlated with increased waist circumference, BMI, and risk of obesity [82]. Studies of prenatal exposure to phthalates and bisphenols have not shown a consistent association with measures of childhood adiposity compared to studies of prenatal exposure to PFAS [83]. Two studies on the American population showed an association between serum concentrations of PFAS and weight gain irrespective of sexes [84]. PFAS, particularly perfluorooctane sulfonate (PFOS) and perfluorononanoic acid (PFNA), were linked with alteration in metabolic rate [85].

Few studies have explored the longitudinal impacts on postnatal growth of prenatal exposure to other chemicals. Evidence risen over the past five years indicates that exposure to phthalates leads to adult weight gain, with most research conducted in women. Some studies by the Women's Health initiative reported a strong correlation between urine concentrations of phthalate metabolites and weight gain [86]. Again, it is to be considered that the effect of a single chemical mostly reflects the epidemiological studies conducted. However, naturally, obesogens ploy cumulative effect as mixtures. The WAT is the depot of obesogens in the human body. More studies should be designed to estimate the accumulative effect of mixtures in future.

6.2 In vitro models

In vitro models have several advantages over other model systems. Taking human cells lines for the study can be of great significance considering the physiological relevance. For screening new chemicals for potential obesogenic properties, in vitro studies are generally conducted before animal models. Several cell lines are used to study the obesogenic impacts of several compounds. Among the in vitro models, mouse embryo pre adipocyte 3 T3-L1 has been used extensively to check the effects of obesogens like TBT [87], BPA [88], BPS [89], genistein [90], phthalate [91], nonylphenol [92] and so on. Other cell lines include C2C12 (mice muscle cells) [93], HELA (human cervical cancer cells) [93], HEK293C (human embryonic kidney cells) [94], HepG2 (human liver carcinoma cells) [95], hASCs (human adipose-derived stem cells) [96], C57BL/6 (mice bone marrow stromal cells) [97], hESCs (human embryonic-derived stem cells) [98] etc.

6.3 In vivo models

Though animal models are not recommended to study certain chemicals' obesogenic potential, they do not mimic the human physiological systems. Still, in vivo model systems have certain advantages over in vitro systems as whole-body kinetics and systemic effects can be studied using animal models. Complex linked pathways involving multiple organs, including adipose tissue, liver, pancreas, muscle, brain, etc., regulate metabolism and weight. In understanding the role of chronic inflammation and hormone interference, in vivo experiment is particularly relevant. The most widely used animal model for the study of obesogens is rodents. Multiple obesogens including TBT [69], BPA [99], triphenyltin [100], DEHP [101], DES [102], polycyclic aromatic hydrocarbons, DDT, and nicotine, have been defined as murine models. Mice are identical biologically and anatomically to humans and share many common diseases. It is incredibly useful for diseases with an inflammatory condition, such as obesity, as animal models can mimic complex inflammatory responses. A transgenic model like obese or lean bodied mice can also be created by manipulating required genes. Other commonly used in vivo models include rats [103], zebrafish [104] and drosophila [105]. Many insights into possible obesogens and various modes of action were provided using in vivo models to investigate endocrine disruption. They may not replicate human physiology, as discussed earlier. Mice exposed to a specified amount of one particular molecule over weeks sometimes does not reflect a chronic variable exposure in humans to multiple chemicals over the years. In detecting obesogens and discerning mechanisms of action, animal models play an essential role. However, they should be combined to draw the most reliable conclusions with knowledge from in vitro studies and epidemiological studies.

7. Strategies for change and future directions

The obesity epidemic first continues in the US and afterwards expands worldwide; therefore, it becomes a dire need to understand the predisposition and related disorders' mechanisms. It becomes of utmost importance to study the extent to which the obesogen exposure influences obesity in humans and establishes the risk factors related to obesity. The risk factors include oxidative stress, inflammation, disrupted circadian rhythms, mitochondrial dysfunction and dietary composition. These interactions may be critical in the effects of obesogen exposure. Evidence documented in the obesogen research area shows that their effect mainly depends on the level and timing of exposure, especially critical windows of exposure during fetal development. Hence, it is crucial to reduce or avoid exposure to obesogens, specifically during pregnancy. However, there is no technique to determine if the individuals have been exposed to any obesogens during their development. It will be a "Holy grail" to identify biomarkers of exposure in obesogen research and establish links among obesogen exposure and other factors related to obesity. The obesogen hypothesis opened a new field into obesity by linking EDCs research with developmental disease origin. The obesogen hypothesis is still in the dearth of research. It requires more studies in the mechanism, developmental time windows and diet interaction. The effects of obesogens are related to epigenetics.

However, we still need more research to understand the mechanism and how the effects get transmitted to forthcoming generations. For instance, how does the obesogen exposure of pregnant Fo female mice lead to obesity in upcoming F3 and F4 unexposed males? There is an extreme lack of data on how obesogen exposure programs adipose tissue dysfunctional that could readily store but not mobilize fat. The obesogen sphere is almost 15 years old only. Much has been studied related to potential effects of EDCs and obesogens. The most substantial evidence for chemical obesogens existence may be the variety of pharmaceuticals that have the side effects of making patients obese. Several international and national workshops have been held to understand the potential role of EDCs in obesity and related metabolic disorders [53]. Thus, various policies and strategies should investigate the magnitude of environmental obesogenic pollutants on the obesity epidemic and the regulatory actions required on such chemicals to improve public health.

8. Conclusion

The majority of evidence that indicates the role of EDCs in driving obesity provides a mechanistic explanation of the obesity epidemic and a management strategy. The role of exogenous chemicals in growing rates of obesity through gene expression regulation (such as PPARs), hormone changes, and inflammation is supported by ample evidence. While overeating, combined with lack of exercise, is undoubtedly a significant contributor to the increase in obesity that can be addressed by decreased calorie intake and increased exercise, it may be that reducing exposure to obesogenic EDCs may also contribute to reducing obesity in the population, especially during the early stages of life. More knowledge of obesogenic pathways will improve prophylactic and therapeutic strategies. The extensive exposure of the human population to so many EDCs with obesogenic action needs evaluation. In vitro models are useful screening devices for detecting and testing obesogenic mechanisms, notably, changes in gene expression or molecular pathways. Improvements to these models will improve human extrapolation in vitro to in vivo as well. However, animal models remain a valuable and typically physiologically precise method for studying obesogenic inter-organ pathways, including hormone interference and inflammation. More epidemiological studies should be made to confirm in vitro and in vivo animal models and provide unparalleled insight into human obesogen exposures and effects. Integrating the data collected from all three of these model systems would result in better-informed choices of compounds that can be used to replace obesogens in food production, packaging, etc. It will, essentially, reduce the economic burden of obesity.

Acknowledgements

All authors thank Banaras Hindu University, India, for providing necessary resources and support to write the present chapter with the support from University Grant Commission (UGC)-Junior Research Fellowship to AM, PG and AS. This work received no external funding from any agency.

Conflict of interest

The author declares that there is no conflict of interest.

Author contributions

All authors listed have made a substantial contribution to this chapter. Moreover, special thanks to PG for writing some sections and proofreading the whole manuscript. Thanks to RKS for reviewing the manuscript before the final submission.

Author details

Archisman Mahapatra, Priya Gupta, Anjali Suman and Rahul Kumar Singh*
Department of Zoology, Molecular Endocrinology and Toxicology Lab (METLab), Institute of Science, Banaras Hindu University, Varanasi, India

*Address all correspondence to: rks.rna@gmail.com

References

[1] EPA, (n.d.). https://www.epa.gov/.

[2] E. Diamanti-Kandarakis, J.-P. Bourguignon, L.C. Giudice, R. Hauser, G.S. Prins, A.M. Soto, R.T. Zoeller, A.C. Gore, Endocrine-disrupting chemicals: an Endocrine Society scientific statement., Endocr. Rev. 30 (2009) 293-342. https://doi.org/10.1210/er.2009-0002.

[3] P. Andrea C. Gore, P. David Crews, P. Loretta L. Doan, M. Michele La Merrill, PhD, P. Heather Patisaul, M. Ami Zota, ScD, INTRODUCTION TO ENDOCRINE DISRUPTING CHEMICALS (EDCs) A GUIDE FOR PUBLIC INTEREST ORGANIZATIONS AND POLICY-MAKERS, Endocr. Soc. (2014).

[4] A.C. Gore, V.A. Chappell, S.E. Fenton, J.A. Flaws, A. Nadal, G.S. Prins, J. Toppari, R.T. Zoeller, EDC-2: The Endocrine Society's Second Scientific Statement on Endocrine-Disrupting Chemicals., Endocr. Rev. 36 (2015) E1–E150. https://doi.org/10.1210/er.2015-1010.

[5] J.J. Heindel, R. Newbold, T.T. Schug, Endocrine disruptors and obesity., Nat. Rev. Endocrinol. 11 (2015) 653-661. https://doi.org/10.1038/nrendo.2015.163.

[6] R.M. Sargis, Metabolic disruption in context: Clinical avenues for synergistic perturbations in energy homeostasis by endocrine disrupting chemicals., Endocr. Disruptors (Austin, Tex.). 3 (2015) e1080788. https://doi.org/10.1080/23273747.2015.1080788.

[7] P. Balaguer, V. Delfosse, M. Grimaldi, W. Bourguet, Structural and functional evidences for the interactions between nuclear hormone receptors and endocrine disruptors at low doses, Comptes Rendus - Biol. 340 (2017) 414-420. https://doi.org/10.1016/j.crvi.2017.08.002.

[8] P.D. Darbre, Endocrine Disruptors and Obesity., Curr. Obes. Rep. 6 (2017) 18-27. https://doi.org/10.1007/s13679-017-0240-4.

[9] R.W. Stahlhut, W. V Welshons, S.H. Swan, Bisphenol A data in NHANES suggest longer than expected half-life, substantial nonfood exposure, or both., Environ. Health Perspect. 117 (2009) 784-789. https://doi.org/10.1289/ehp.0800376.

[10] A.M. Calafat, X. Ye, L.-Y. Wong, J.A. Reidy, L.L. Needham, Exposure of the US population to bisphenol A and 4-tertiary-octylphenol: 2003-2004., Environ. Health Perspect. 116 (2008) 39-44. https://doi.org/10.1289/ehp.10753.

[11] C. Casals-Casas, B. Desvergne, Endocrine disruptors: from endocrine to metabolic disruption., Annu. Rev. Physiol. 73 (2011) 135-162. https://doi.org/10.1146/annurev-physiol-012110-142200.

[12] F. Grün, B. Blumberg, Perturbed nuclear receptor signaling by environmental obesogens as emerging factors in the obesity crisis., Rev. Endocr. Metab. Disord. 8 (2007) 161-171. https://doi.org/10.1007/s11154-007-9049-x.

[13] A. Janesick, B. Blumberg, Minireview: PPARγ as the target of obesogens., J. Steroid Biochem. Mol. Biol. 127 (2011) 4-8. https://doi.org/10.1016/j.jsbmb.2011.01.005.

[14] M. Chandra, S. Miriyala, M. Panchatcharam, PPARγ and Its Role in Cardiovascular Diseases., PPAR Res. 2017 (2017) 6404638. https://doi.org/10.1155/2017/6404638.

[15] R.T. Zoeller, Environmental chemicals impacting the thyroid: targets and consequences., Thyroid. 17 (2007) 811-817. https://doi.org/10.1089/thy.2007.0107.

[16] M. Boas, K.M. Main, U. Feldt-Rasmussen, Environmental chemicals

and thyroid function: an update., Curr. Opin. Endocrinol. Diabetes. Obes. 16 (2009) 385-391. https://doi.org/10.1097/MED.0b013e3283305af7.

[17] WHO, WHO report, (n.d.). https://www.who.int/news-room/fact-sheets/detail/obesity-and-overweight.

[18] CDC, About adult BMI, (2017). https://www.cdc.gov/healthyweight/assessing/bmi/adult_bmi/index.html.

[19] S. Wan Siang Cheong, Gen Re, Overweight and Obesity in Asia, Underwrit. Focus. (2014).

[20] J.J. Heindel, B. Blumberg, Environmental Obesogens: Mechanisms and Controversies., Annu. Rev. Pharmacol. Toxicol. 59 (2019) 89-106. https://doi.org/10.1146/annurev-pharmtox-010818-021304.

[21] L.N. Vandenberg, T. Colborn, T.B. Hayes, J.J. Heindel, D.R.J. Jacobs, D.-H. Lee, T. Shioda, A.M. Soto, F.S. vom Saal, W. V Welshons, R.T. Zoeller, J.P. Myers, Hormones and endocrine-disrupting chemicals: low-dose effects and nonmonotonic dose responses., Endocr. Rev. 33 (2012) 378-455. https://doi.org/10.1210/er.2011-1050.

[22] P.M. Schlosser, Inhalation Exposure and Absorption of Toxicants, Compr. Toxicol. (2010) 75.

[23] H. Cumming, C. Rücker, Octanol-Water Partition Coefficient Measurement by a Simple (1)H NMR Method., ACS Omega. 2 (2017) 6244-6249. https://doi.org/10.1021/acsomega.7b01102.

[24] E. Jackson, R. Shoemaker, N. Larian, L. Cassis, Adipose Tissue as a Site of Toxin Accumulation, Compr. Physiol. (2017) 1085-1135. https://doi.org/https://doi.org/10.1002/cphy.c160038.

[25] Y.-M. Lee, K.-S. Kim, D.R.J. Jacobs, D.-H. Lee, Persistent organic pollutants in adipose tissue should be considered in obesity research., Obes. Rev. an Off. J. Int. Assoc. Study Obes. 18 (2017) 129-139. https://doi.org/10.1111/obr.12481.

[26] H. Choudhury, T. Harvey, W.C. Thayer, T.F. Lockwood, W.M. Stiteler, P.E. Goodrum, J.M. Hassett, G.L. Diamond, Urinary cadmium elimination as a biomarker of exposure for evaluating a cadmium dietary exposure--biokinetics model., J. Toxicol. Environ. Health. A. 63 (2001) 321-350. https://doi.org/10.1080/15287390152103643.

[27] J. Oh, J.W. Choi, Y.-A. Ahn, S. Kim, Pharmacokinetics of bisphenol S in humans after single oral administration., Environ. Int. 112 (2018) 127-133. https://doi.org/10.1016/j.envint.2017.11.020.

[28] H. Liu, S. Tang, X. Zheng, Y. Zhu, Z. Ma, C. Liu, M. Hecker, DM V Saunders, J.P. Giesy, X. Zhang, H. Yu, Bioaccumulation, biotransformation, and toxicity of BDE-47, 6-OH-BDE-47, and 6-MeO-BDE-47 in early life-stages of zebrafish (*Danio rerio*)., Environ. Sci. Technol. 49 (2015) 1823-1833. https://doi.org/10.1021/es503833q.

[29] D.F. Staskal, J.J. Diliberto, M.J. DeVito, L.S. Birnbaum, Toxicokinetics of BDE 47 in female mice: effect of dose, route of exposure, and time., Toxicol. Sci. 83 (2005) 215-223. https://doi.org/10.1093/toxsci/kfi018.

[30] M.O. Milbrath, Y. Wenger, C.-W. Chang, C. Emond, D. Garabrant, B.W. Gillespie, O. Jolliet, Apparent half-lives of dioxins, furans, and polychlorinated biphenyls as a function of age, body fat, smoking status, and breast-feeding., Environ. Health Perspect. 117 (2009) 417-425. https://doi.org/10.1289/ehp.11781.

[31] PubChem, https://pubchem.ncbi.nlm.nih.gov/compound/Bis_2-ethylhexyl_-phthalate, (n.d.). https://pubchem.ncbi.nlm.nih.gov/compound/Bis_2-ethylhexyl_-phthalate.

[32] L. Magos, W. J. Hayes, Jr. and E. R. Laws, Jr. Handbook of pesticide toxicology volume 1: General principles; Volumes 2 and 3: Classes of pesticides. Academic Press, San Diego, 1991. 1576 pp., $395.00, J. Appl. Toxicol. 12 (1992) 75-76. https://doi.org/https://doi.org/10.1002/jat.2550120118.

[33] T. Woodruff, M.S. Wolff, D.L. Davis, D. Hayward, Organochlorine exposure estimation in the study of cancer etiology., Environ. Res. 65 (1994) 132-144. https://doi.org/10.1006/enrs.1994.1026.

[34] European Commission, 2005.

[35] International Programme on Chemical Safety as accessed on 8 Feb, 2021, (n.d.). http://www.inchem.org/documents/pims/chemical/pimg018.htm.

[36] USD of H. And, H. Services, PH Service, A. for T. Substances, and D. Registry, ToxGuideTM for Atrazine, 2003.

[37] C.E. Reed, S.E. Fenton, Exposure to diethylstilbestrol during sensitive life stages: a legacy of heritable health effects., Birth Defects Res. C. Embryo Today. 99 (2013) 134-146. https://doi.org/10.1002/bdrc.21035.

[38] International Programme on Chemical Safety as accessed on 8 Feb, 2021, (n.d.). http://www.inchem.org/documents/pims/chemical/nicotine.htm.

[39] P. Tontonoz, B.M. Spiegelman, Fat and beyond: the diverse biology of PPARgamma., Annu. Rev. Biochem. 77 (2008) 289-312. https://doi.org/10.1146/annurev.biochem.77.061307.091829.

[40] F. Grün, H. Watanabe, Z. Zamanian, L. Maeda, K. Arima, R. Cubacha, D.M. Gardiner, J. Kanno, T. Iguchi, B. Blumberg, Endocrine-disrupting organotin compounds are potent inducers of adipogenesis in vertebrates., Mol. Endocrinol. 20 (2006) 2141-2155. https://doi.org/10.1210/me.2005-0367.

[41] A. le Maire, M. Grimaldi, D. Roecklin, S. Dagnino, V. Vivat-Hannah, P. Balaguer, W. Bourguet, Activation of RXR-PPAR heterodimers by organotin environmental endocrine disruptors., EMBO Rep. 10 (2009) 367-373. https://doi.org/10.1038/embor.2009.8.

[42] L. Yin, K.S. Yu, K. Lu, X. Yu, Benzyl butyl phthalate promotes adipogenesis in 3T3-L1 preadipocytes: A High Content Cellomics and metabolomic analysis., Toxicol. In Vitro. 32 (2016) 297-309. https://doi.org/10.1016/j.tiv.2016.01.010.

[43] S. Kirchner, T. Kieu, C. Chow, S. Casey, B. Blumberg, Prenatal exposure to the environmental obesogen tributyltin predisposes multipotent stem cells to become adipocytes., Mol. Endocrinol. 24 (2010) 526-539. https://doi.org/10.1210/me.2009-0261.

[44] X. Li, J. Ycaza, B. Blumberg, The environmental obesogen tributyltin chloride acts via peroxisome proliferator activated receptor gamma to induce adipogenesis in murine 3T3-L1 preadipocytes., J. Steroid Biochem. Mol. Biol. 127 (2011) 9-15. https://doi.org/10.1016/j.jsbmb.2011.03.012.

[45] H. Masuno, T. Kidani, K. Sekiya, K. Sakayama, T. Shiosaka, H. Yamamoto, K. Honda, Bisphenol A in combination with insulin can accelerate the conversion of 3T3-L1 fibroblasts to adipocytes., J. Lipid Res. 43 (2002) 676-684.

[46] M. Penza, C. Montani, A. Romani, P. Vignolini, B. Pampaloni, A. Tanini, M.L. Brandi, P. Alonso-Magdalena, A. Nadal, L. Ottobrini, O. Parolini, E. Bignotti, S. Calza, A. Maggi, P.G. Grigolato, D. Di Lorenzo, Genistein affects adipose tissue deposition in a dose-dependent and gender-specific manner., Endocrinology. 147 (2006) 5740-5751. https://doi.org/10.1210/en.2006-0365.

[47] S.A. Whitehead, S. Rice, Endocrine-disrupting chemicals as modulators of sex steroid synthesis., Best Pract. Res. Clin. Endocrinol. Metab. 20 (2006) 45-61. https://doi.org/10.1016/j.beem.2005.09.003.

[48] G. Williams, Aromatase up-regulation, insulin and raised intracellular oestrogens in men, induce adiposity, metabolic syndrome and prostate disease, via aberrant ER-α and GPER signalling., Mol. Cell. Endocrinol. 351 (2012) 269-278. https://doi.org/10.1016/j.mce.2011.12.017.

[49] BM. Shoucri, B. Blumberg, Impact of Environmental Obesogens, Child. Obes. (2016) 219-234. https://doi.org/10.1201/9781315370958-21.

[50] S. Ho, W. Tang, Techniques used in studies of epigenome dysregulation due to aberrant DNA methylation: an emphasis on fetal-based adult diseases., Reprod. Toxicol. 23 (2007) 267-282. https://doi.org/10.1016/j.reprotox.2007.01.004.

[51] T.T. Schug, A. Janesick, B. Blumberg, J.J. Heindel, Endocrine disrupting chemicals and disease susceptibility, J. Steroid Biochem. Mol. Biol. 127 (2011) 204-215. https://doi.org/10.1016/j.jsbmb.2011.08.007.

[52] A. Nadal, I. Quesada, E. Tudurí, R. Nogueiras, P. Alonso-Magdalena, Endocrine-disrupting chemicals and the regulation of energy balance, Nat. Rev. Endocrinol. 13 (2017) 536-546. https://doi.org/10.1038/nrendo.2017.51.

[53] M.K. Lee, B. Blumberg, Transgenerational effects of obesogens, Basic Clin. Pharmacol. Toxicol. 125 (2019) 44-57. https://doi.org/https://doi.org/10.1111/bcpt.13214.

[54] P.J. Turnbaugh, F. Bäckhed, L. Fulton, J.I. Gordon, Diet-induced obesity is linked to marked but reversible alterations in the mouse distal gut microbiome., Cell Host Microbe. 3 (2008) 213-223. https://doi.org/10.1016/j.chom.2008.02.015.

[55] P.J. Turnbaugh, R.E. Ley, M.A. Mahowald, V. Magrini, E.R. Mardis, J.I. Gordon, An obesity-associated gut microbiome with increased capacity for energy harvest., Nature. 444 (2006) 1027-1031. https://doi.org/10.1038/nature05414.

[56] A. Vrieze, E. Van Nood, F. Holleman, J. Salojärvi, R.S. Kootte, J.F.W.M. Bartelsman, G.M. Dallinga-Thie, M.T. Ackermans, M.J. Serlie, R. Oozeer, M. Derrien, A. Druesne, J.E.T. Van Hylckama Vlieg, V.W. Bloks, A.K. Groen, H.G.H.J. Heilig, E.G. Zoetendal, E.S. Stroes, W.M. de Vos, J.B.L. Hoekstra, M. Nieuwdorp, Transfer of intestinal microbiota from lean donors increases insulin sensitivity in individuals with metabolic syndrome., Gastroenterology. 143 (2012) 913-6.e7. https://doi.org/10.1053/j.gastro.2012.06.031.

[57] A.N. Buerger, D.T. Dillon, J. Schmidt, T. Yang, J. Zubcevic, C.J. Martyniuk, J.H.J. Bisesi, Gastrointestinal dysbiosis following diethylhexyl phthalate exposure in zebrafish (Danio rerio): Altered microbial diversity, functionality, and network connectivity., Environ. Pollut. 265 (2020) 114496. https://doi.org/10.1016/j.envpol.2020.114496.

[58] J. Zhan, X. Ma, D. Liu, Y. Liang, P. Li, J. Cui, Z. Zhou, P. Wang, Gut microbiome alterations induced by tributyltin exposure are associated with increased body weight, impaired glucose and insulin homeostasis and endocrine disruption in mice., Environ. Pollut. 266 (2020) 115276. https://doi.org/10.1016/j.envpol.2020.115276.

[59] K.-P. Lai, Y.-T. Chung, R. Li, H.-T. Wan, C.K.-C. Wong, Bisphenol A alters gut microbiome: Comparative metagenomics analysis., Environ. Pollut. 218 (2016) 923-930. https://doi.org/10.1016/j.envpol.2016.08.039.

[60] U.-H. Jin, S.-O. Lee, G. Sridharan, K. Lee, L.A. Davidson, A. Jayaraman, R.S. Chapkin, R. Alaniz, S. Safe, Microbiome-derived tryptophan metabolites and their aryl hydrocarbon receptor-dependent agonist and antagonist activities., Mol. Pharmacol. 85 (2014) 777-788. https://doi.org/10.1124/mol.113.091165.

[61] J. Ji, H. Qu, Cross-regulatory Circuit Between AHR and Microbiota., Curr. Drug Metab. 20 (2019) 4-8. https://doi.org/10.2174/1389200219666180129151150.

[62] B. Chassaing, O. Koren, J.K. Goodrich, A.C. Poole, S. Srinivasan, R.E. Ley, A.T. Gewirtz, Dietary emulsifiers impact the mouse gut microbiota promoting colitis and metabolic syndrome., Nature. 519 (2015) 92-96. https://doi.org/10.1038/nature14232.

[63] A. Mahapatra, P. Gupta, R.K. Singh, An Overview of Sars-Cov-2 Features, Replication, Pathophysiology and Therapeutic Approaches, COVID-19 Pandemic Updat. 2020. (2020) 29-53. https://doi.org/10.26524/royal.37.3.

[64] Y. Cui, Z.-F. Zhang, J. Froines, J. Zhao, H. Wang, S.-Z. Yu, R. Detels, Air pollution and case fatality of SARS in the People's Republic of China: an ecologic study., Environ. Health. 2 (2003) 15. https://doi.org/10.1186/1476-069X-2-15.

[65] F. Nappi, L. Barrea, C. Di Somma, M.C. Savanelli, G. Muscogiuri, F. Orio, S. Savastano, Endocrine Aspects of Environmental "Obesogen" Pollutants., Int. J. Environ. Res. Public Health. 13 (2016). https://doi.org/10.3390/ijerph13080765.

[66] J.S. Kim, Z. Chen, T.L. Alderete, C. Toledo-Corral, F. Lurmann, K. Berhane, F.D. Gilliland, Associations of air pollution, obesity and cardiometabolic health in young adults: The Meta-AIR study., Environ. Int. 133 (2019) 105180. https://doi.org/10.1016/j.envint.2019.105180.

[67] Z. Zheng, X. Xu, X. Zhang, A. Wang, C. Zhang, M. Hüttemann, L.I. Grossman, L.C. Chen, S. Rajagopalan, Q. Sun, K. Zhang, Exposure to ambient particulate matter induces a NASH-like phenotype and impairs hepatic glucose metabolism in an animal model., J. Hepatol. 58 (2013) 148-154. https://doi.org/10.1016/j.jhep.2012.08.009.

[68] MD. Anway, A.S. Cupp, M. Uzumcu, M.K. Skinner, Epigenetic transgenerational actions of endocrine disruptors and male fertility., Science. 308 (2005) 1466-1469. https://doi.org/10.1126/science.1108190.

[69] R. Chamorro-García, M. Sahu, R.J. Abbey, J. Laude, N. Pham, B. Blumberg, Transgenerational inheritance of increased fat depot size, stem cell reprogramming, and hepatic steatosis elicited by prenatal exposure to the obesogen tributyltin in mice., Environ. Health Perspect. 121 (2013) 359-366. https://doi.org/10.1289/ehp.1205701.

[70] M. Manikkam, R. Tracey, C. Guerrero-Bosagna, M.K. Skinner, Plastics derived endocrine disruptors (BPA, DEHP and DBP) induce epigenetic transgenerational inheritance of obesity, reproductive disease and sperm epimutations., PLoS One. 8 (2013) e55387. https://doi.org/10.1371/journal.pone.0055387.

[71] M. Manikkam, M.M. Haque, C. Guerrero-Bosagna, E.E. Nilsson, M.K. Skinner, Pesticide methoxychlor promotes the epigenetic transgenerational inheritance of adult-onset disease through the female germline., PLoS One. 9 (2014) e102091. https://doi.org/10.1371/journal.pone.0102091.

[72] R. Tracey, M. Manikkam, C. Guerrero-Bosagna, M.K. Skinner, Hydrocarbons (jet fuel JP-8) induce epigenetic transgenerational inheritance

of obesity, reproductive disease and sperm epimutations., Reprod. Toxicol. 36 (2013) 104-116. https://doi.org/10.1016/j.reprotox.2012.11.011.

[73] M.K. Skinner, M. Manikkam, R. Tracey, C. Guerrero-Bosagna, M. Haque, E.E. Nilsson, Ancestral dichlorodiphenyltrichloroethane (DDT) exposure promotes epigenetic transgenerational inheritance of obesity, BMC Med. 11 (2013) 228. https://doi.org/10.1186/1741-7015-11-228.

[74] E. Whitelaw, Disputing Lamarckian epigenetic inheritance in mammals., Genome Biol. 16 (2015) 60. https://doi.org/10.1186/s13059-015-0626-0.

[75] A.P. Starling, J.L. Adgate, R.F. Hamman, K. Kechris, A.M. Calafat, D. Dabelea, Prenatal exposure to per- and polyfluoroalkyl substances and infant growth and adiposity: the Healthy Start Study., Environ. Int. 131 (2019) 104983. https://doi.org/10.1016/j.envint.2019.104983.

[76] TI. Halldorsson, D. Rytter, L.S. Haug, B.H. Bech, I. Danielsen, G. Becher, T.B. Henriksen, S.F. Olsen, Prenatal exposure to perfluorooctanoate and risk of overweight at 20 years of age: a prospective cohort study., Environ. Health Perspect. 120 (2012) 668-673. https://doi.org/10.1289/ehp.1104034.

[77] J.M. Braun, A. Chen, ME Romano, A.M. Calafat, G.M. Webster, K. Yolton, B.P. Lanphear, Prenatal perfluoroalkyl substance exposure and child adiposity at 8 years of age: The HOME study., Obesity (Silver Spring). 24 (2016) 231-237. https://doi.org/10.1002/oby.21258.

[78] T.J. Hartman, A.M. Calafat, A.K. Holmes, M. Marcus, K. Northstone, W.D. Flanders, K. Kato, E. V Taylor, Prenatal Exposure to Perfluoroalkyl Substances and Body Fatness in Girls., Child. Obes. 13 (2017) 222-230. https://doi.org/10.1089/chi.2016.0126.

[79] A.M. Mora, E. Oken, S.L. Rifas-Shiman, T.F. Webster, M.W. Gillman, A.M. Calafat, X. Ye, S.K. Sagiv, Prenatal Exposure to Perfluoroalkyl Substances and Adiposity in Early and Mid-Childhood., Environ. Health Perspect. 125 (2017) 467-473. https://doi.org/10.1289/EHP246.

[80] P. Liu, F. Yang, Y. Wang, Z. Yuan, Perfluorooctanoic Acid (PFOA) Exposure in Early Life Increases Risk of Childhood Adiposity: A Meta-Analysis of Prospective Cohort Studies., Int. J. Environ. Res. Public Health. 15 (2018). https://doi.org/10.3390/ijerph15102070.

[81] J.P. Buckley, S.M. Engel, J.M. Braun, R.M. Whyatt, J.L. Daniels, M.A. Mendez, D.B. Richardson, Y. Xu, A.M. Calafat, M.S. Wolff, B.P. Lanphear, A.H. Herring, A.G. Rundle, Prenatal Phthalate Exposures and Body Mass Index Among 4- to 7-Year-old Children: A Pooled Analysis., Epidemiology. 27 (2016) 449-458. https://doi.org/10.1097/EDE.0000000000000436.

[82] D. Valvi, M. Casas, M.A. Mendez, A. Ballesteros-Gómez, N. Luque, S. Rubio, J. Sunyer, M. Vrijheid, Prenatal bisphenol a urine concentrations and early rapid growth and overweight risk in the offspring., Epidemiology. 24 (2013) 791-799. https://doi.org/10.1097/EDE.0b013e3182a67822.

[83] L.G. Kahn, C. Philippat, S.F. Nakayama, R. Slama, L. Trasande, Endocrine-disrupting chemicals: implications for human health., Lancet. Diabetes Endocrinol. 8 (2020) 703-718. https://doi.org/10.1016/S2213-8587(20)30129-7.

[84] B.E. Blake, S.M. Pinney, E.P. Hines, S.E. Fenton, K.K. Ferguson, Associations between longitudinal serum perfluoroalkyl substance (PFAS) levels and measures of thyroid hormone, kidney function, and body mass index in the Fernald Community Cohort., Environ. Pollut. 242 (2018)

894-904. https://doi.org/10.1016/j.envpol.2018.07.042.

[85] G. Liu, K. Dhana, J.D. Furtado, J. Rood, G. Zong, L. Liang, L. Qi, G.A. Bray, L. DeJonge, B. Coull, P. Grandjean, Q. Sun, Perfluoroalkyl substances and changes in body weight and resting metabolic rate in response to weight-loss diets: A prospective study., PLoS Med. 15 (2018) e1002502. https://doi.org/10.1371/journal.pmed.1002502.

[86] M. V Díaz Santana, S.E. Hankinson, C. Bigelow, S.R. Sturgeon, R.T. Zoeller, L. Tinker, J.A.E. Manson, A.M. Calafat, J.R. Meliker, K.W. Reeves, Urinary concentrations of phthalate biomarkers and weight change among postmenopausal women: a prospective cohort study., Environ. Health. 18 (2019) 20. https://doi.org/10.1186/s12940-019-0458-6.

[87] A. Pereira-Fernandes, C. Vanparys, T.L.M. Hectors, L. Vergauwen, D. Knapen, P.G. Jorens, R. Blust, Unraveling the mode of action of an obesogen: mechanistic analysis of the model obesogen tributyltin in the 3T3-L1 cell line., Mol. Cell. Endocrinol. 370 (2013) 52-64. https://doi.org/10.1016/j.mce.2013.02.011.

[88] F. Ariemma, V. D'Esposito, D. Liguoro, F. Oriente, S. Cabaro, A. Liotti, I. Cimmino, M. Longo, F. Beguinot, P. Formisano, R. Valentino, Low-Dose Bisphenol-A Impairs Adipogenesis and Generates Dysfunctional 3T3-L1 Adipocytes., PLoS One. 11 (2016) e0150762. https://doi.org/10.1371/journal.pone.0150762.

[89] M.Á. Martínez, J. Blanco, J. Rovira, V. Kumar, J.L. Domingo, M. Schuhmacher, Bisphenol A analogues (BPS and BPF) present a greater obesogenic capacity in 3T3-L1 cell line., Food Chem. Toxicol. an Int. J. Publ. Br. Ind. Biol. Res. Assoc. 140 (2020) 111298. https://doi.org/10.1016/j.fct.2020.111298.

[90] J.E. Davis, D. Hastings, Transcriptional Regulation of TCF/LEF and PPARγ by Daidzein and Genistein in 3T3-L1 Preadipocytes., J. Med. Food. 21 (2018) 761-768. https://doi.org/10.1089/jmf.2017.0136.

[91] W. Qi, Q. Xu, Y. Xu, Z. Wang, L. Yang, S. Guo, Y. Shi, T. Zhao, L. Zhou, L. Ye, Effect of Notch pathway on lipid accumulation induced by mono-2-ethylhexyl phthalate on 3T3-L1 cells., Ecotoxicol. Environ. Saf. 208 (2021) 111472. https://doi.org/10.1016/j.ecoenv.2020.111472.

[92] H. Masuno, S. Okamoto, J. Iwanami, K. Honda, T. Shiosaka, T. Kidani, K. Sakayama, H. Yamamoto, Effect of 4-nonylphenol on cell proliferation and adipocyte formation in cultures of fully differentiated 3T3-L1 cells., Toxicol. Sci. 75 (2003) 314-320. https://doi.org/10.1093/toxsci/kfg203.

[93] C.H. Hurst, D.J. Waxman, Activation of PPARalpha and PPARgamma by environmental phthalate monoesters., Toxicol. Sci. 74 (2003) 297-308. https://doi.org/10.1093/toxsci/kfg145.

[94] A.M. Temkin, R.R. Bowers, M.E. Magaletta, S. Holshouser, A. Maggi, P. Ciana, L.J. Guillette, J.A. Bowden, J.R. Kucklick, J.E. Baatz, DD. Spyropoulos, Effects of Crude Oil/Dispersant Mixture and Dispersant Components on PPARγ Activity in Vitro and in Vivo: Identification of Dioctyl Sodium Sulfosuccinate (DOSS; CAS #577-11-7) as a Probable Obesogen., Environ. Health Perspect. 124 (2016) 112-119. https://doi.org/10.1289/ehp.1409672.

[95] Z. Sun, H. Cao, Q.S. Liu, Y. Liang, H. Fiedler, J. Zhang, Q. Zhou, G. Jiang, 4-Hexylphenol influences adipogenic differentiation and hepatic lipid accumulation in vitro., Environ. Pollut. 268 (2021) 115635. https://doi.org/10.1016/j.envpol.2020.115635.

[96] J.K. Hartman, T. Beames, B. Parks, D. Doheny, G. Song, A. Efremenko,

M. Yoon, B. Foley, C. Deisenroth, P.D. McMullen, R.A. Clewell, An in vitro approach for prioritization and evaluation of chemical effects on glucocorticoid receptor mediated adipogenesis., Toxicol. Appl. Pharmacol. 355 (2018) 112-126. https://doi.org/10.1016/j.taap.2018.05.016.

[97] L. Ivry Del Moral, L. Le Corre, H. Poirier, I. Niot, T. Truntzer, J.-F. Merlin, P. Rouimi, P. Besnard, R. Rahmani, M.C. Chagnon, Obesogen effects after perinatal exposure of 4,4′-sulfonyldiphenol (Bisphenol S) in C57BL/6 mice., Toxicology. 357-358 (2016) 11-20. https://doi.org/10.1016/j.tox.2016.05.023.

[98] R.Y. Wang, R.D. Abbott, A. Zieba, F.E. Borowsky, D.L. Kaplan, Development of a Three-Dimensional Adipose Tissue Model for Studying Embryonic Exposures to Obesogenic Chemicals., Ann. Biomed. Eng. 45 (2017) 1807-1818. https://doi.org/10.1007/s10439-016-1752-x.

[99] A. Brulport, D. Vaiman, M.-C. Chagnon, L. Le Corre, Obesogen effect of bisphenol S alters mRNA expression and DNA methylation profiling in male mouse liver., Chemosphere. 241 (2020) 125092. https://doi.org/10.1016/j.chemosphere.2019.125092.

[100] J. Watt, J.J. Schlezinger, Structurally diverse, PPARγ-activating environmental toxicants induce adipogenesis and suppress osteogenesis in bone marrow mesenchymal stromal cells., Toxicology. 331 (2015) 66-77. https://doi.org/10.1016/j.tox.2015.03.006.

[101] Y. Yang, F. Sun, H. Chen, H. Tan, L. Yang, L. Zhang, J. Xie, J. Sun, X. Huang, Y. Huang, Postnatal exposure to DINP was associated with greater alterations of lipidomic markers for hepatic steatosis than DEHP in postweaning mice., Sci. Total Environ. 758 (2021) 143631. https://doi.org/10.1016/j.scitotenv.2020.143631.

[102] T.O. Owuor, M. Reid, L. Reschke, I. Hagemann, S. Greco, Z. Modi, K.H. Moley, Maternal obesogenic diet induces endometrial hyperplasia, an early hallmark of endometrial cancer, in a diethylstilbestrol mouse model., PLoS One. 13 (2018) e0186390. https://doi.org/10.1371/journal.pone.0186390.

[103] J.F.P. de Araújo, P.L. Podratz, G.C. Sena, E. Merlo, L.C. Freitas-Lima, J.G.M. Ayub, A.F.Z. Pereira, A.P. Santos-Silva, L. Miranda-Alves, I. V Silva, J.B. Graceli, The obesogen tributyltin induces abnormal ovarian adipogenesis in adult female rats., Toxicol. Lett. 295 (2018) 99-114. https://doi.org/10.1016/j.toxlet.2018.06.1068.

[104] A. Lyssimachou, J.G. Santos, A. André, J. Soares, D. Lima, L. Guimarães, C.M.R. Almeida, C. Teixeira, L.F.C. Castro, M.M. Santos, The Mammalian "Obesogen" Tributyltin Targets Hepatic Triglyceride Accumulation and the Transcriptional Regulation of Lipid Metabolism in the Liver and Brain of Zebrafish., PLoS One. 10 (2015) e0143911. https://doi.org/10.1371/journal.pone.0143911.

[105] Z. Yu, J. Shen, Z. Li, J. Yao, W. Li, L. Xue, L.N. Vandenberg, D. Yin, Obesogenic Effect of Sulfamethoxazole on *Drosophila melanogaster* with Simultaneous Disturbances on Eclosion Rhythm, Glucolipid Metabolism, and Microbiota., Environ. Sci. Technol. 54 (2020) 5667-5675. https://doi.org/10.1021/acs.est.9b07889.

Chapter 4

Critical Analysis of Human Exposure to Bisphenol A and Its Novel Implications on Renal, Cardiovascular and Hypertensive Diseases

Rafael Moreno-Gómez-Toledano, María I. Arenas, Sandra Sánchez-Esteban, Alberto Cook, Marta Saura and Ricardo J. Bosch

Abstract

Bisphenol A (BPA), an endocrine disruptor involved in synthesizing numerous types of plastics, is detected in almost the entire population's urine. The present work aims to estimate daily exposure to BPA by systematically reviewing all articles with original data related to urinary BPA concentration. This approach is based on human pharmacokinetic models, which have shown that 100% of BPA (free and metabolized form) is eliminated only in a few hours through urine. Several extensive population studies and experimental data have recently proven a significant association between urinary excretion of BPA and albuminuria, associated with renal damage. Our team's previous work has shown that low-dose BPA can promote a cytotoxic effect on renal mouse podocytes. Moreover, BPA administration in mice promotes kidney damage and hypertension. Furthermore, preliminary studies in human renal cells in culture (podocytes) strongly suggest that BPA might also promote kidney damage. Overall, the present review analyzed BPA exposure data from mammalian cell studies, experimental animal models, and several human populations. Studying principal cohorts calculated the exposures to BPA globally, showing a high BPA exposure suggesting the need to decrease BPA exposure more effectively, emphasizing groups with higher sensitivity as kidney disease patients.

Keywords: bisphenol A, systematic review, human, urine, estimated daily intake

1. Introduction: brief historical overview

Bisphenol A is the perfect example of the double edge of industrial development. On the one hand, thanks to BPA, we have countless plastic objects with excellent physical properties at low prices; on the other hand, increasing exposure to this kind of xenobiotic compounds could be a severe health risk to the general population.

BPA is a phenolic compound widely distributed due to its multiple uses as an additive and plasticizer in plastic polymers' manufacture [1]. This compound can be found in various everyday items, such as food containers, toys, dental supplies, electronic devices, and even clothing [2–6].

The BPA problem presents a particular and curious situation: BPA is a compound whose properties as an estrogen modulator were already determined 84 years ago by medical researchers at the University of London [7], but its use increased substantially last decades. The discoverer's idea was to commercialize a compound that could treat female pathologies. Finally, they succeeded with Diethylstilbestrol, a substance with much greater potency than BPA, and was introduced in the 1940s [8].

It took about 50 years since the Russian chemist Dianin synthesized it in 1891 [9, 10] until the BPA began to be used in the industrial manufacturing of epoxy resins. Still, due to its incredible versatility, BPA quickly achieved great importance in the American industry. In the mid-1970s, the BPA was considered a part, directly or indirectly, of all major US industries [8]. In parallel, Schnell's contributions in 1956 demonstrated BPA's potential role in producing polycarbonates [11, 12]. Due to its unique combination of physical properties, this type of compound has had a significant impact on the world industry, as have epoxy resins. Today they are still used in numerous applications, such as in the automotive or LED sector [12]. In fact, there is a tendency to increase its consumption in the coming years, as can be seen in the Asian market, where there has been a substantial increase in the demand for polycarbonates in the last ten years [13]. It is expected to continue growing in the years to come, as observed in the American market [14].

2. Novel role of BPA in renal, cardiovascular and hypertensive diseases; latest discoveries

2.1 BPA in the renal system

BPA is a compound widely studied for its estrogenic properties within the field of fertility and sexual organs. However, other organs, such as the kidney and liver, may have the highest exposure ranges. In the kidney's case, BPA concentration has been positively correlated with a greater predisposition to kidney pathologies [15–17] or clinical signs associated with kidney diseases, such as increased albuminuria or decreased glomerular filtration rate [18–21].

Our group has worked on BPA's possible action on the renal system in recent years, using different cell and animal models. The first steps were carried out on a renal cell line of immortalized mouse podocytes. It was possible to observe how the chronic treatment of BPA exerts a cytotoxic effect on the cells. The administration of 10 and 100 nM doses for nine days exerted loss of cell viability and increased apoptosis (as assessed by MTT and TUNEL, respectively). These effects were accompanied by an increase in the synthesis of molecules classically involved in the pathogenesis of glomerulosclerosis, such as the cyclin-dependent kinase inhibitor p27kip1, the TGF-β system, and collagen IV. Furthermore, in these cells, BPA reduced the synthesis of nephrin and podocin, proteins of the filtration slits involved in proteinuria and podocyte survival mechanisms. As would be expected from these in vitro results, the kidneys of animals treated with BPA developed hypertrophy, hyperfiltration, and proteinuria. Along with the increased renal expression of p27kip1, TGF-β, and collagen IV, mesangial expansion and a decrease in the number of podocytes due to apoptosis were also seen. Electron microscopy showed hypertrophy of podocytes and pedicles. It should be noted that even when animals treated with BPA did not develop hyperglycaemia, their kidneys showed structural and functional changes similar to those that occur in the initial stages of diabetic nephropathy (DN) (**Figure 1**) [22, 23].

Secondly, the possible effects of BPA on an immortalized human podocyte cell line were explored. We observed that BPA promotes a novel type of podocytopathy characterized by an impairment of cell adhesion by altering adhesion and cytoskeleton proteins' expression.

By using transcriptomics, proteomics, western-blot, and immunocytochemistry, it was possible to determine that BPA at low doses promotes a reduction in the expression of numerous structural or adhesion proteins, such as tubulin, vimentin, podocin, cofilin-1, vinculin, E-cadherin, nephrin, and VCAM-1, as well as an increase in the expression of proteins that negatively participate in adhesion mechanisms, such as Tenascin-C [24].

Since podocytes do not replicate in adults, the resulting podocytopenia after the urinary loss of podocytes might promote glomerulosclerosis. Collectively all available data suggest that BPA could participate in the pathogenesis and progression of renal diseases. It is essential to mention that these experimental results are supported by epidemiological studies conducted in the populations of New York [25], Shanghai [19],

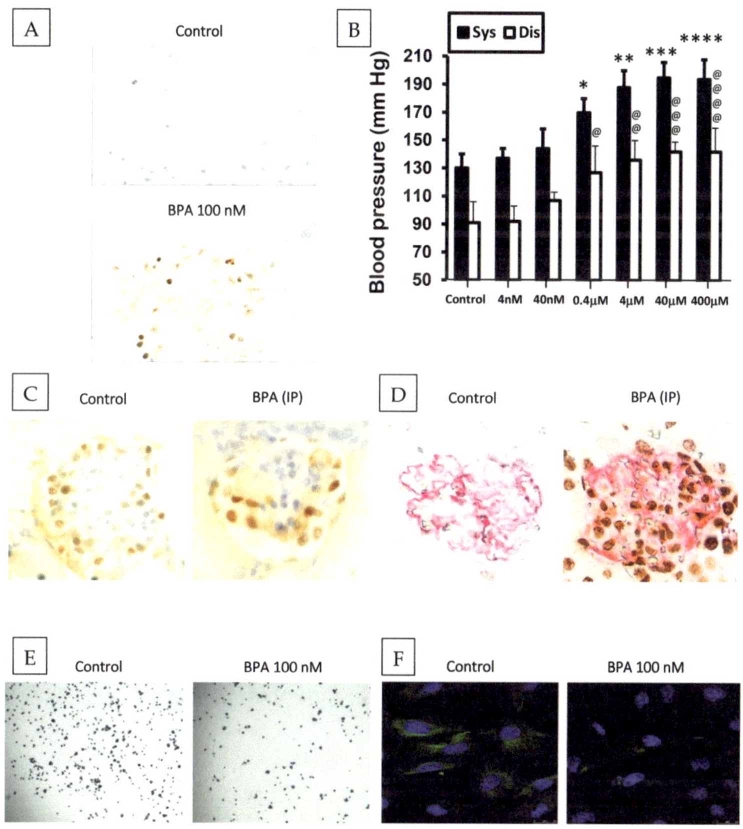

Figure 1.
*Notable evidence from cell and animal models. A) TUNEL technique performed in mouse podocytes. Note the significant increase in the number of apoptotic cells in the cells treated with BPA. B) Hypertensive effect of BPA administered to animals in drinking water. C) Reduction in the number of glomerular podocytes (labelled with WT-1) of the mice treated with intraperitoneal (IP) BPA. D) Increased number of apoptotic kidney cells (TUNEL) of mice treated with IP BPA. E) Adhesion assay in human podocytes. A reduction of up to 50% was observed in cells treated with BPA. F) Podocin immunocytochemistry in human podocytes. A significant loss of labelling is evidenced in cells treated with BPA. * or @ means p-value < 0,05; ** or @@ means p < 0,01; *** or @@@ means p < 0,001; **** or @@@@ means p < 0,0001. Figure made with our own results published in the Journal of Cellular Physiology [22], FASEB Journal [27] and Scientific Reports [24].*

and Seoul [26], which describe an association between human exposure to BPA and an increase in proteinuria and hypertension.

2.2 BPA in the cardiovascular system

Further studies demonstrated that animals treated with BPA developed arterial hypertension and endothelial dysfunction in a dose-dependent manner (**Figure 1**). Microarray analysis of gene expression in murine endothelial cells treated with BPA demonstrated the activation of genes involved in vascular regulation, such as angiotensin II and calcium-calmodulin kinase II (CaMKII). This event was subsequently observed in vivo as well. The activation is responsible for the endothelial dysfunction and hypertension induced by BPA, given that CaMKII activation promotes the enzymatic uncoupling of endothelial nitric oxide synthase. This phenomenon leads to oxygen free radicals' production instead of nitric oxide, a primary vasodilator, and endothelial protector. Moreover, this increased production of oxygen free radicals indicates that BPA, and inducing hypertension, could participate in vascular damage mechanisms and atherosclerotic lesions' progression [23, 27]. Besides, recent data demonstrated the cardiotoxic effect of BPA by a mechanism that involved activation of the RIP 3-CamKII necroptotic pathway leading to endothelial cell death. Decreased endothelial barrier function and weakening of the coronary vascular wall in the setting of hypertension may cause ventricular hemorrhages, cardiac and lung congestion, which ultimately led to heart failure [28].

3. BPA exposure in the general population. Identification of groups with higher exposure

3.1 Pharmacokinetics of BPA

The heterogeneous distribution of BPA results in the ability to enter the body in multiple ways. The main entry route is considered oral, through the ingestion of food or beverages containing BPA [29, 30]. However, there are other routes like inhalation (air or dust) [31–34], dermal (cosmetics, thermal tickets) [35–37], and it has even been hypothesized with the ocular [38] and sublingual routes [35, 39]. It is estimated that between 85 and 100% of the BPA ingested can be absorbed through the intestine. Thanks to its capacity to cross biological barriers, it has been observed that BPA has the potential to distribute itself through any fluid and biological tissue, even crossing the transplacental or blood–brain barrier [29, 40, 41]. In the case of the dermal route, it has been determined that the ability of BPA to enter the body is lower, with percentages less than 10% [42, 43]. For its part, the sublingual route (of great importance in the elements used in dentistry) seems that it could become more efficient than the intestinal entry [39].

BPA's metabolism is marked by phase II reactions, biochemical mechanisms capable of modifying its structure to facilitate its excretion [44]. BPA is metabolized towards glucuronidation or sulfonation in the intestine and the liver [41, 45, 46], but the metabolic capacity can be seriously reduced in diseases such as obesity or diabetes [47]. Glucuronidation is the majority reaction, mediated by uridine diphosphate glucuronosyltransferase (UGT) [44, 48]. It has also been suggested that a part of the BPA that reaches the intestine could be degraded to p-cresol by the intestinal microbiota, thus generating uremic toxins [49]. Another possible route studied has been hydroxylation to catechol, followed by a transformation to o-quinone. This route, like the previous one, can generate toxicity associated with oxidative stress [50].

Pharmacokinetic studies in rodents have determined that BPA is excreted in urine and feces [29, 51, 52]. It has been observed that BPA is excreted exclusively through the urine in non-human primates and humans [41, 53, 54]. This phenomenon makes it much easier to make a rough estimate of the degree of exposure by BPA's urinary quantification. The inter-species differences observed are attributed to a possible higher enterohepatic recirculation in rodents [29, 51, 52]. However, there is evidence that contradicts this hypothesis [55].

3.2 Calculation of BPA exposure in the general population

As mentioned above, thanks to pharmacokinetic studies in humans [41, 53, 54], it is accepted that 100% of BPA is eliminated via the urinary tract, which can be used to determine the degree of daily exposure to this compound quickly. For this reason, we proceed to evaluate the question of the degree of global exposure through a systematic review of principal cohorts in the world. To estimate human exposure to BPA, we first collected data published by one of the world's largest cohorts: the National Health and Nutrition Examination Survey (NHANES). NHANES is a survey research program conducted by the US National Center for Health Statistics (NCHS), with more than 72,000 patients studied between 2003 and 2016 [56].

After extracting all the data and unifying them, 18,244 urinary BPA concentrations were obtained. A non-parametric distribution was obtained after performing

Continent	N	Population group (cohort / city)	GM
America	18,244	General population [Own study*]	1.77
Asia	6,003	General Population (KoNEHS) [57]	1.13
America	5,476	General Population (CHMS) [58]	1.6
Asia	3,455	General Population (Shanghai) [19]	0.82
Asia	2,535	Pregnant (Wuhan) [59]	0.9
America	2,477	General Population (Ex-R study) [60]	1.96
America	2,318	General Population (HOPE) [61]	2.52
Asia	2,044	General Population (KRIEFS) [62]	1.83
Europe	1,996	Pregnant (SELMA) [63]	1.53
America	1,933	Pregnant (MIREC) [64]	0.9
America	1,868	Pregnant (PROTECT) [65]	2.02
Europe	1,764	Pregnant (Elfe) [66]	0.69
Asia	1,625	General Population (KEEP) [67]	0.71
America	1,543	Pregnant (LifeCodes) [68]	1.18
Europe	1,396	Pregnant (Generation R) [69]	1.68
Europe	1,146	General Population (DESIR) [70]	1.78
Europe	1,084	Pregnant (HELIX) [71]	3.38
Oceania	420	General Population (Brisbane) [72]	2.61
Africa	210	General Population (Giza) [73]	0.68

Note that two results have been included with a reduced sample size to include Oceania and Africa. Meaning of abbreviations: K, kids; A, adults; GM, geometric mean (or corrected median).
**Own study corresponds with NHANES 2003 – 2016 cohort.*

Table 1.
Representative data from the main cohorts in the world.

the normality tests, for which the geometric mean (GM) was calculated, obtaining a result of 1.77 ng/ml. A systematic review of urinary BPA was then carried out to select from among all the publications with the most representative cohorts from each continent and the largest number of people. Using the keywords: Bisphenol AND (urine OR urinary) in the reference search engines Pubmed and Web of Science, a total of 999 and 2,025 results were obtained, respectively. Once the duplicates were eliminated, a total of 2,414 publications remained. After screening by title/abstract, a total of 756 publications were selected. Finally, after reading in-depth, 447 articles were selected whose pages describe urinary concentrations of BPA in some population groups, either general or specific, such as patients with various pathologies, pregnant women, the elderly, or workers subjected to occupational exposure. All data from the 447 academic articles were collected and analyzed carefully. According to the country, population group, and sample size, the primary world cohorts were selected from all of them, obtaining 16 cohorts whose sample sizes exceed 1000 individuals from America, Asia, and Europe (**Table 1**). A result of Oceania and another from Australia was also included due to representability. All of them expressed the concentration of BPA in ng/ml except one of them, which expressed it in μg per gram of creatinine (μg/g creat.) [71]. Therefore, it was modified by calculating the average creatinine concentration in adults using the NHANES cohort's data and the other two major cohorts, KoNEHS and CHMS [74, 75].

We consider that in the study of urinary BPA, where the results follow non-parametric distributions, the values that should be analyzed would correspond to the GM or the median. To determine if both values can be unified, they were examined using linear regression, observing that they were always in the same range, and the variation between them was relatively small. The equation of a line was **$Y = 0.9855 * X$, and $R^2 = 0.9919$**. For this reason, the decision was reached to

Country	N	Population	GM	Units	nM
Iran	132	Gen.Pop. [76]	232.6	ng/ml	1,018.88
China	74	Oc.Exp. [77]	199.13	μg/g creat.	872.27
China	72	Oc.Exp. [78]	158.41	μg/g creat.	693.9
USA	525	Oc.Exp. [79]	107	ng/ml	468.7
Country	**N**	**Population**	**Median**	**Units**	**nM**
China	72	Oc.Exp. [78]	238.78	μg/g creat.	1,045.95
China	74	Oc.Exp. [77]	180.59	μg/g creat.	791.06
USA	525	Oc.Exp. [79]	108	ng/ml	473.08
China	198	Oc.Exp. [80]	84.6	μg/g creat.	370.58
Country	**N**	**Population**	**P95**	**Units**	**nM**
China	74	Oc.Exp. [77]	23,979.51	μg/g creat.	105,039.69
USA	112	Pregnant [81]	250.06	ng/ml	1,095.36
France	254	Pregnant [82]	115.4	ng/ml	505.5
Belgium	72	ICU patients [83]	113.7	ng/ml	498.05
Country	**N**	**Population**	**MAX**	**Units**	**nM**
China	74	Oc.Exp. [77]	264,219.38	μg/g creat.	1,157,384.82
USA	525	Oc.Exp. [79]	32,900	ng/ml	144,114.94
China	28	Oc.Exp. [84]	1,934.85	ng/ml	8,475.4
France	390	Oc.Exp. [85]	1,915	ng/ml	8,388.45

Meaning of abbreviations: Gen.Pop., General population; Oc.Exp., Occupational Exposure.

Table 2.
Higher urinary BPA values determined according to the geometric mean (GM), median, 95th percentile (P95), or maximum value (MAX).

use the GM, preferably, but if it was not recorded, use the median corrected with the equation obtained.

Next, the urinary BPA was averaged, considering each cohort's sample size, obtaining a final result of **1.55 ng/ml** (with a sample size of 57,537 individuals). Once the average concentration determined in the general population's urine has been established, the next step will be carried out on the highest values found in the systematic review to determine interest groups to study BPA exposure.

As reflected in **Table 2**, it is clear that workers subjected to occupational exposure are the ones who are likely to find a more significant entry of BPA into their bodies. The highest values observed, both of the median and the maximum value (MAX), correspond entirely to people subjected to occupational exposure, such as workers in the plastics industry. The highest GM value stands out, as it corresponds to the general Iranian population. An in-depth study would be necessary to be able to discern the problem that underlies this study area. Interestingly, unusually high 95th percentile values can also be seen in pregnant women and intensive care patients. It is likely that consumable medical supplies, such as catheters or hemodialyzers, could increase BPA exposure due to their plastic composition. Bearing this in mind, and in keeping with the discoveries described in basic research, the study and analysis of BPA exposure in patients undergoing hemodialysis is crucial.

4. Systematic review of BPA exposure in hemodialysis patients

After describing the latest advances in the BPA-kidney paradigm investigation, the need to include kidney patients as a group of special vulnerability to exposure to BPA is evident. Thereof, there is a point of convergence in the final stages within the different pathologies or stages: the need for dialysis due to the kidney's reduced functionality. Interestingly, there is evidence that the use of surgical medical equipment can increase exposure to compounds such as BPA due to the composition of its materials. Therefore, we will analyze the urinary concentration of BPA in patients undergoing hemodialysis procedures to estimate the daily exposure to which they are subjected. The systematic review methodology was used again, using the keywords: bisphenol AND (dialysis OR hemodialyzer OR hemodiafiltration OR hemodialysis OR dialyzer).

Thirty-eight results were obtained in Pubmed and 50 in Web of Science. After eliminating duplicates, a total of 66 documents were obtained. Once the first screening by title/abstract was done to look for BPA concentrations in patients undergoing hemodialysis, a total of 20 publications were accepted. After carefully studying the text, ten publications were selected[1]. Of these, only 1 quantifies the urinary BPA concentration in dialysis patients [87] and 9 in serum [15, 86–94].

The publication by Schöringhumer et al., which quantifies urinary BPA, obtains concentrations between 0.4 and 2.6 ng/ml within the same range as the general population [87], equivalent to 1.75–11.39 nM. In general terms, low exposure would be considered. Still, considering the in vitro model results and the patient's pathology, it could pose an added risk for kidney disease evolution. In the case of publications that study BPA in serum, some show values similar to those observed in the general population's urine. Among them, we can find the publications of Kanno et al. (5.3 ± 0.3 ng/ml), Murakami et al. (values between 1.48 ± 1.41 and 6.62 ± 3.09), Sajiki et al. (values between 0.179 ± 0.263 and 0.642 ± 1.443), Shen et al. (1.01) or Turgut et al. (5.57 ± 1.2) [88, 90, 92–94]. Higher values have the publications of Quiroga et al. (high flux hemodialysis: 7.5 ± 3.5; online hemodiafiltration: 6.7 ± 2.5)

[1] Those publications without relevant data, reviews, and conference communications were discarded.

and Krieter et al. (10 ± 6.6) [15, 91]. Finally, Bosch-Panadero et al. and Mas et al. describe serum BPA values in patients undergoing conventional dialysis that range from 52.73 ± 60.6 to 163.03 ± 155.84. Also, they quantify serum BPA concentrations in patients undergoing online hemodiafiltration from 8.79 ± 7.97 to 23.42 ± 20.38) [86, 89]. These high values would be equivalent to 230.98–714.14 nM in the case of conventional dialysis and 38.50–102.59 nM in online hemodiafiltration.

5. Systematic review of occupational exposure to BPA

The alarming data described in the previous pages denote the need to study occupational exposure. To this end, we proceeded to use two academic reference search engines, Pubmed and Web of Science, using the following keywords: Bisphenol AND (workers OR occupational exposure OR exposure workplace), obtaining a total of 658 publications (once repeated results were eliminated). Of all of them, 25 publications were adapted to the search. Only publications with urinary BPA (or blood) concentrations were selected in workers with high exposure or themselves before and after their work shift. Of the 25 studies selected for their affinity with the topic of interest, we can distinguish three subgroups: In the first (G1)[2], BPA concentrations can be observed well above the average, and with significant differences between the study groups. In the second group (G2)[3], there are concentrations higher than the mean in a range closer to it, while in the third group (G3), the range of concentrations is within the range of values of the general population.

5.1 G1: extremely high BPA concentrations

From a quantitative perspective, within G1, the most interesting publication is Liu et al. [95]. It compares BPA concentrations in people with potential occupational exposure versus controls, obtaining substantially different values. The median values (interquartile range, IR) between exposed workers vs. controls are 685.9 (43.7–3671.8) vs. 4.2 (0–15.9) μg/g creat. Other equally interesting values are Tian et al. [78] and Song et al. [77]. Firstly, they determine geometric mean (GM) values (standard deviation, SD) between exposed subjects vs. control of 158.41 (17.92) vs. 0.84 (6.53) μg/g creat., reaching in the second publication, the values of 199.13 (19.65) vs. 0.77 (6.33) μg/g creat. Song et al.'s publication determine the highest maximum urinary BPA concentration, reaching the value of 264,219.38 μg/g creat., (264.22 mg/g creat.).

The next publications to consider are two by Hines et al. [79, 96], where they study exposure to BPA in different factories before and after the work shift. In them, essential differences can be appreciated, showing, to cite an example of each article, a GM (SD) in pre-shift vs. post-shift of 6.2 (4.3) vs. 130 (10) μg/sample or 26.6 (5.74) vs. 178 (6.2) μg/g creat. These groups show arithmetic mean (SD) values of 15 (22) vs. 2300 (5800) μg/sample and 115 (252) vs. 812 (2330) μg/g creat. The maximum BPA value is also very striking, reaching 32,900 ng/ml. We will continue with the study of publications with high BPA values, Xiao et al. [97], and the two publications by Li et al. [98, 99]. They show differences between exposed workers vs. control, showing medians of 101.94 vs. 0 ng/ml of serum in the first case and

[2] All those publications with geometric means or medians greater than 50 (ng/ml, μg/g creat., μg/urine sample, or ng/ml of plasma) have been selected.

[3] We have selected those publications with values of geometric means/medians lower than 50 and higher than 8 (at least four times above the global mean).

57.9 vs. 1.2 and 53.7 vs. 1.2 μg/g in the other two. Finally, it is important to mention the works of He et al. [80] and Wang et al. [84]. In the first, they find pre-shift vs. post-shift differences of 84.6 vs. 111 μg/g creat. (median) and 4630 vs. 5400 μg/g creat. (AM). In the second publication, they quantify urinary BPA concentrations in workers of an epoxy resin factory, with a GM (SD) of 55.73 (5.48) and a maximum value of 1934.85 ng/ml.

5.2 G2: elevated BPA concentrations

Within G2, where the concentrations are not so high, articles such as those by Li et al. [100] or Miao et al. [101, 102]. In them, differences between exposed vs. control are determined, observing medians (IR) of 38.7 (6.3–354.3) vs. 1.4 (0.0–17.9) μg/g creat. in the first case, AM (SD) of 36.23 (7.69) vs. 1.38 (6.89) μg/g creat. in the second, and GM (95% confidence interval, CI) of 22.2 (12.4–39.8) vs. 0.9 (0.7–1.1) μg/g creat. in the latter. The same pattern can be observed in the work of Ndaw et al. [85], where higher values are observed in cashiers exposed to thermal tickets vs. controls, determining a GM (SD) of 8.58 (2.83) vs. 3.52 (2.35). For their part, Zhuang et al. [103] carried out a slightly different approach since they determined differences between workers of an epoxy resin company with a working time greater than five years versus those in the company for less than five years. The median values observed reflected a significant increase in workers with a longer working time (27.18 vs. 9.73 ng/ml serum). Finally, the work of Heinälä et al. [104] is also included in this group, where the pre-shift vs. post-shift urinary concentration is studied, quantitatively highlighting the GM of the heat-sensitive paper producing company, 18.7 vs. 39.4 ng/ml, or from the liquid paint producer, 4.6 vs. 10.3 ng/ml of urine.

5.3 G3: "normal" range but with significant differences

The third group, G3, despite being in the range that we have determined as general, corresponding to the majority of the population, also presents interesting differences. Among them, the works of Zhou et al. [105] and Kouidhi et al. [106] stand out. Their comparison between exposed subjects vs. controls found values corresponding to the median of 3.198 vs. 0.276 ng/ml serum in the first and 3.81 vs. 0.73 ng/ml urine in the second. The same study line is the oldest academic article of the review, published by Hanaoka et al. in 2002 [107]. They determined very few differences between workers in the bisphenol diglycidyl ether (BADGE) industry vs. controls, with medians of 1.06 vs. 0.52 μmol/mol creat. Similarly, He et al. [108] determine few differences between exposed workers and their families, determining a GM of 1.41 ng/ml in exposed men, compared to 0.58 in their women or 0.78 in their children under 20 years of age. Waldman et al. [109] and González et al. [110] also show low GM values. The first measures BPA's urinary concentrations in firefighters, engineers, captains, or battalion commanders, determining a GM of 1.58 ng/ml. In the second, they determine BPA's concentration in workers of an incinerator of hazardous waste, determining a GM of 0.68 in men and 1.2 ng/ml in women. Thayer et al. [111] and Lee et al. [36] carried out two publications focusing on cashiers exposed to thermal tickets. The first determines GM (SD) in pre-shift vs. post-shift cashiers of 1.89 (3.63) vs. 2.76 (3.53) μg/g creat., being 1.25 (1.79) in controls that do not work as cashiers. The second publication finds subtle differences only in those cashiers who do not wear gloves, observing GM values pre- vs. post-shift of 0.4 vs. 0.9 ng/ml in cashiers without gloves, and 0.44 vs. 0.49 ng/ml in tellers with gloves. Finally, it remains to mention the work of Hehn et al. [112], in which analyzing the data from the American health program NHANES according to the possible potential exposure. They determine GM values in women with probable vs. unlikely exposure of 5.45 vs. 2.16 ng/ml, thus as of 2.85 vs. 2.59 ng/ml in men's case.

6. Tolerable daily intake (TDI); calculations and extrapolations

Tolerable Daily Intake (TDI) is "the maximum amount of a contaminant which can be eaten every day over a whole lifetime without incurring appreciable risk to health" [113]. Currently, the European Food Safety Authority (EFSA) estimates it at 4 μg/kg BW/day [31]. The TDI calculated by EFSA is based on the studies of Tyl et al. [114], in which the concentration limit at which no adverse effects were observed, NOEL or NOAEL, was determined. They used concentrations from 0.03 to 50 and 600 mg/kg BW/day (0.018–3500 ppm) in mice of different generations. They only observed renal effects (increase in organ weight) at the highest dose (600 mg/kg BW/day), thereby determining the NOEL at the next lower dose they used, which corresponds to 50 mg/kg BW/day. Thus, based on the renal NOEL/NOAEL and due to the presumption of limitations in the use of the parameter, the EFSA calculates the equivalent "Benchmark dose" (BMD). The equivalent concentration, in which it is estimated that there is an alteration in kidney weight in 10% of the treated animals, is 9 mg/kg. After applying a correction factor to estimate the equivalent dose in humans, a concentration of about 600 μg/kg is obtained. Finally, an uncertainty factor of 150 is applied to obtain the final result of 4 μg/kg BW/day [31].

To determine if the population is exposed to a high or low BPA concentration, the estimated daily intake (EDI) must finally be calculated. Exposure levels are expressed as a mass (nanograms or micrograms) per kg of weight per day. For this reason, it is necessary to multiply the urinary concentration of BPA in ng/ml by the average volume of urine (in ml) excreted per day and divide this number by the average weight measured in kilograms (reference values extracted from academic literature [115]). When taking the average value between adult men and women, a value of 1400 ml per day is obtained. The publication itself also shows the reference values for body weight, expressed in kg. When taking the same average as that applied to the urinary volume, adults' average weight would correspond to a value of 66.5 kg. In this way, as reflected in **Table 3**, the main EDIs were calculated.

Statistical parameter	Population	Value (ng/ml)	μg/kg BW/day
GM	General population [own work]	1.55	0.03
AM	Conventional dialysis [86]	52.73 to 155.84	1.11 – 3.28
AM	Online hemodiafiltration [86]	8.79 to 23.42	0.19 – 0.49
Median	Occupational Exposure [78]	243.08	5.12
MAX	Occupational Exposure [77]	268,975.33	5.662.64
P95	Pregnant woman [81]	250.06	5.26
P95	ICU patients [83]	113.7	2.39

Note that the maximum occupational exposure value reaches 5.66 mg/kg BW/day (1000 times higher than TDI). Abbreviations: GM, geometric mean; AM, arithmetic mean; MAX, maximum value; P95, 95th percentile.

Table 3.
Most relevant values in the systematic review.

7. Discussion

In the first place, an interesting element to consider resides in the pharmacokinetics models since they add modifications to BPA in order to determine it efficiently and without contamination by HPLC. After the first model made by Volkel et al. [41], where they used d(16)-bisphenol A, successive authors have emulated this methodology in order to accurately measure the pharmacokinetics of administered BPA [54, 55, 116–119]. However, deuterium modification of drugs is used today to reduce toxicity by redirecting metabolic pathways [120]. Perhaps the possibility that not all BPA is excreted in urine should be reconsidered with this in mind. We know that mice excrete BPA in feces; however, there are no publications in the literature that quantify BPA in human feces, although the presence of microplastics in them has recently been demonstrated [121].

Secondly, since it is described that BPA is a hydrophobic molecule, but with slight aqueous solubility and with the capacity to cross all types of biological tissues [29, 41, 122], it is possible their bioaccumulation in the organism. To do this, Richard W. Stahlhut's team determined BPA concentrations as a function of fasting time. Surprisingly, BPA levels did not decrease rapidly with fasting time, suggesting that there may be non-food exposure or bioaccumulation in body tissues [123].

Thirdly, another critical element is the possible non-monotonic effects of BPA on various organs and tissues [124–126]. This non-monotonicity can significantly affect at low concentrations, below the current TDI, in the same way that it has been shown to happen with certain hormonal stimuli. In her review, Vanderberg [124] determined that non-monotonic dose–response curves (NMDRCs) are typical in the literature related to BPA, occurring in greater than 20% of all experiments and at least one endpoint in more than 30% of all studies examined [124]. Going a little deeper into the non-monotonic effects works such as that of Angle et al. demonstrate the existence of multimodal dose–response curves [127]. Recent data suggest that the non-monotonic effect of BPA could depend upon the target tissue. In our studies in mice, we observed that while BPA induces hypertension in a dose-dependent manner, it affects renal podocytes in a classical non-monotonic response curve [22, 23, 27]. In multimodal curves, increases and decreases are observed, and variations in the maximum response depending on the type of tissue [127] may further complicate the correct assessment of BPA's presumed safety concentrations currently found in the population.

Throughout this chapter, an average urinary BPA value for the general population has been determined using a systematic methodology to serve as a reference. Similarly, the analysis of the different statistical parameters shown in the publications determined population groups of special interest, such as workers with occupational exposure, pregnant women, or intensive care patients. With the latest discoveries in the BPA-nephro-vascular system paradigm, all this provides a sufficient basis to place kidney patients in the critical spotlight. The systematic review has determined relatively high BPA plasma values in patients undergoing hemodialysis, which could be a potentiating element for its worsening. In this way, the need to modify the materials used in specific treatments to reduce exposure to this endocrine disruptor is determined, thus avoiding some patients' possible deterioration. Similarly, the high values of urinary BPA in various publications related to occupational exposure show the need to improve personal protective equipment and working conditions in specific sectors related to the manufacture or recycling of plastics, since concentrations should not be detected urinary levels high enough to reach the micromolar or even nanomolar range. Although we have indeed normalized the existence of endocrine disruptors in the general population's urine, which is a worrying fact, we should ensure that they are at the lowest possible threshold.

EFSA determines that the TDI is at four μg/kg BW/day, which is justified with experimental animal models. However, as in vitro experiments have shown, BPA can exert very different actions in murine and human cells, although with similar consequences, converging on the possibility of kidney damage. It remains to be determined whether it would be necessary to review the coherence of the calculations and extrapolations, taking into account the observed inter-species differences.

8. Conclusions

- Novel data suggest that human exposure to bisphenol A is associated with renal, cardiovascular, and hypertensive diseases.

- The inter-species differences observed in the basic research models show interesting evidence to rethink the institutions' calculations that determine the TDI.

- The use of modified molecules in the pharmacokinetic models and the absence of studies in feces (and the presence of microplastics) suggest the possibility that not all BPA is excreted in the urine, which would mean that the concentrations described would be below the actual exposure.

- The development of the systematic review using the premise of pharmacokinetic studies shows a relatively low general exposure, but with population groups of interest, such as workers with occupational exposure and patients from the hospital environment.

- The data obtained and the novelties in basic research provide sufficient evidence to consider the patient with kidney disease as one of the priority groups in which their exposure should be reduced, possibly by modifying the medical material's composition.

Acknowledgements

This work was supported in part by grants from Instituto de Salud Carlos III (PI15/02,139) -Fondo Europeo de Desarrollo Regional (FEDER)-.

R. Moreno- Gómez-Toledano is recipient of a research contract from CAM (B2017-BMD-3686).

Author details

Rafael Moreno-Gómez-Toledano[1], María I. Arenas[3], Sandra Sánchez-Esteban[2], Alberto Cook[2], Marta Saura[2] and Ricardo J. Bosch[1*]

1 Laboratory of Renal Physiology and Experimental Nephrology, University of Alcalá, Alcalá de Henares, SPAIN

2 Laboratory of Pathophysiology of the Vascular Wall, Department of System Biology/Physiology Unit, University of Alcalá, Alcalá de Henares, SPAIN

3 Department of Biomedicine and Biotechnology/Cell Biology Unit, University of Alcalá, Alcalá de Henares, SPAIN

*Address all correspondence to: ricardoj.bosch@uah.es

References

[1] Thomas S, Visakh P (eds). *Handbook of Engineering and Specialty Thermoplastics, Volume 3: Polyethers and Polyesters*. Wiley, 2011.

[2] Vandenberg LN, Hauser R, Marcus M, et al. Human exposure to bisphenol A (BPA). *Reprod Toxicol* 2007; 24: 139-177.

[3] Ministerio de Medio Ambiente y Medio Rural y Marino (MARM). *Mejores Técnicas Disponibles de referencia europea. Producción de Polímeros.* Madrid, 2009.

[4] Dursun E, Fron-Chabouis H, Attal J-P, et al. Bisphenol A Release: Survey of the Composition of Dental Composite Resins. *Open Dent J* 2016; 10: 446-453.

[5] Li AJ, Kannan K. Elevated Concentrations of Bisphenols, Benzophenones, and Antimicrobials in Pantyhose Collected from Six Countries. *Environ Sci Technol* 2018; 52: 10812-10819.

[6] Freire C, Molina-Molina JM, Iribarne-Durán LM, et al. Concentrations of bisphenol A and parabens in socks for infants and young children in Spain and their hormone-like activities. *Environ Int* 2019; 127: 592-600.

[7] Dodds EC, Lawson W. Synthetic Estrogenic agents without phenanthrene nucleus. *Nature* 1936; 137: 996.

[8] Vogel SA. The politics of plastics: the making and unmaking of bisphenol a 'safety'. *Am J Public Health* 2009; 99 Suppl 3: S559–S566.

[9] Rubin BSBS. Bisphenol A: An endocrine disruptor with widespread exposure and multiple effects. *J Steroid Biochem Mol Biol* 2011; 127: 27-34.

[10] Rutkowska A, Rachoń D. Bisphenol A (BPA) and its potential role in the pathogenesis of the polycystic ovary syndrome (PCOS). *Gynecol Endocrinol* 2014; 30: 260-265.

[11] Feldman D. Polymer history. *Des Monomers Polym* 2008; 11: 1-15.

[12] Olabisi O, Adewale K. Handbook of Thermoplastics, Second Edition. *Plast Eng* 2016; 41: 1003.

[13] Jiang D, Chen WQ, Liu W, et al. Inter-Sectoral Bisphenol A (BPA) Flows in the 2012 Chinese Economy. *Environ Sci Technol* 2017; 51: 8654-8662.

[14] Grand View Research. Polycarbonate Sheet Market Size & Share | Industry Report, 2018-2025, https://www.grandviewresearch.com/industry-analysis/polycarbonate-sheet-market (2018, accessed 11 September 2020).

[15] Krieter DH, Canaud B, Lemke H-D, et al. Bisphenol A in chronic kidney disease. *Artif Organs* 2013; 37: 283-290.

[16] Hu J, Yang S, Wang Y, et al. Serum bisphenol A and progression of type 2 diabetic nephropathy: a 6-year prospective study. *ACTA Diabetol* 2015; 52: 1135-1141.

[17] Hu J, Wang Y, Xiang X, et al. Serum bisphenol A as a predictor of chronic kidney disease progression in primary hypertension: a 6-year prospective study. *J Hypertens* 2016; 34: 332-337.

[18] You L, Zhu X, Shrubsole MJ, et al. Renal function, bisphenol A, and alkylphenols: Results from the National Health and Nutrition Examination Survey (NHANES 2003-2006). *Environ Health Perspect* 2011; 119: 527-533.

[19] Li M, Bi Y, Qi L, et al. Exposure to bisphenol A is associated with low-grade albuminuria in Chinese adults. *Kidney Int* 2012; 81: 1131-1139.

[20] Trasande L, Attina TM, Trachtman H. Bisphenol A exposure is associated with low-grade urinary albumin excretion in children of the United States. *Kidney Int* 2013; 83: 741-748.

[21] Kang H, Kim S, Lee G, et al. Urinary metabolites of dibutyl phthalate and benzophenone-3 are potential chemical risk factors of chronic kidney function markers among healthy women. *Environ Int* 2019; 124: 354-360.

[22] Olea-Herrero N, Arenas MIMI, Muñóz-Moreno C, et al. Bisphenol-A induces podocytopathy with proteinuria in mice. *J Cell Physiol* 2014; 229: 2057-2066.

[23] Bosch RJ, Quiroga B, Munoz-Moreno C, et al. Bisphenol A: An environmental factor implicated in renal vascular damage. *Nefrologia : publicacion oficial de la Sociedad Espanola Nefrologia* 2016; 36: 5-9.

[24] Moreno-Gómez-Toledano R, Arenas MI, González-Martínez C, et al. Bisphenol A impaired cell adhesion by altering the expression of adhesion and cytoskeleton proteins on human podocytes. *Sci Rep* 2020; 10: 16638.

[25] Trasande L, Sathyanarayana S, Trachtman H. Dietary phthalates and low-grade albuminuria in US children and adolescents. *Clin J Am Soc Nephrol* 2014; 9: 100-109.

[26] Bae S, Hong Y-C. Exposure to bisphenol A from drinking canned beverages increases blood pressure: randomized crossover trial. *Hypertens (Dallas, Tex 1979)* 2015; 65: 313-319.

[27] Saura M, Marquez S, Reventun P, et al. Oral administration of bisphenol A induces high blood pressure through angiotensin II/CaMKII-dependent uncoupling of eNOS. *FASEB J*; 28. Epub ahead of print 2014. DOI: 10.1096/fj.14-252460.

[28] Reventun P, Sanchez-Esteban S, Cook A, et al. Bisphenol A induces coronary endothelial cell necroptosis by activating RIP3/CamKII dependent pathway. *Sci Rep*; 10. Epub ahead of print 1 December 2020. DOI: 10.1038/s41598-020-61014-1.

[29] FAO/WHO Expert Meeting and Stakeholder Meeting on Bisphenol A Food and Agriculture Organization of the United Nations. *Toxicological and Health Aspects of Bisphenol A*. Ottawa, Canada, www.who.int (2010, accessed 4 April 2019).

[30] Rudel RA, Gray JM, Engel CL, et al. Food Packaging and Bisphenol A and Bis(2-Ethyhexyl) Phthalate Exposure: Findings from a Dietary Intervention. *Environ Health Perspect* 2011; 119: 914-920.

[31] EFSA Panel on Food Contact Materials Enzymes Flavourings and Processing Aids. Scientific Opinion on the risks to public health related to the presence of bisphenol A (BPA) in foodstuffs. *EFSA J* 2016; 13: 3978.

[32] Ruiz Montes A. *Evaluación de la exposición a Bisfenol-A en población infantil de la provincia de Granada, e identificación de factores asociados*. Universidad de Granada, 2010.

[33] Konieczna A, Rutkowska A, Rachoń D. Health risk of exposure to Bisphenol A (BPA). *Rocz Panstw Zakl Hig* 2015; 66: 5-11.

[34] Robinson L, Miller R. The Impact of Bisphenol A and Phthalates on Allergy, Asthma, and Immune Function: a Review of Latest Findings. *Current environmental health reports* 2015; 2: 379-387.

[35] Hormann AM, Vom Saal FS, Nagel SC, et al. Holding thermal receipt paper and eating food after using hand sanitizer results in high serum bioactive

and urine total levels of bisphenol A (BPA). *PLoS One* 2014; 9: e110509.

[36] Lee I, Kim S, Kim KT, et al. Bisphenol A exposure through receipt handling and its association with insulin resistance among female cashiers. *Environ Int* 2018; 117: 268-275.

[37] Liu J, Martin JW. Prolonged Exposure to Bisphenol A from Single Dermal Contact Events. *Environ Sci Technol* 2017; 51: 9940-9949.

[38] Mas S, Egido J, González-Parra E, et al. Importancia del bisfenol A, una toxina urémica de origen exógeno, en el paciente en hemodiálisis. *Nefrología* 2017; 37: 229-234.

[39] Gayrard V, Lacroix MZ, Collet SH, et al. High bioavailability of bisphenol A from sublingual exposure. *Environ Health Perspect* 2013; 121: 951-956.

[40] Vandenberg LN, Chahoud I, Heindel JJ, et al. Urinary, Circulating, and Tissue Biomonitoring Studies Indicate Widespread Exposure to Bisphenol A (vol 118, pg 1055, 2010). *Cien Saude Colet* 2012; 17: 809.

[41] Volkel W, Colnot T, Csanady GA, et al. Metabolism and kinetics of bisphenol a in humans at low doses following oral administration. *Chem Res Toxicol* 2002; 15: 1281-1287.

[42] Demierre A-LL, Peter R, Oberli A, et al. Dermal penetration of bisphenol A in human skin contributes marginally to total exposure. *Toxicol Lett* 2012; 213: 305-308.

[43] Instituto Nacional de Seguriad e Higiene en el Trabajo. *Bisfenol A Documentación toxicológica para el establecimiento del límite de exposición*, http://www.insht.es/InshtWeb/Contenidos/Documentacion/LEP _ VALORES LIMITE/Doc_Toxicologica/Ficheros 2011/DLEP 60 Bisfenol A.pdf (2011, accessed 4 April 2019).

[44] Teeguarden JG, Calafat AM, Ye X, et al. Twenty-Four Hour Human Urine and Serum Profiles of Bisphenol A during High-Dietary Exposure. *Toxicol Sci* 2011; 123: 48-57.

[45] Teeguarden JG, Waechter JM, Clewell HJ, et al. Evaluation of oral and intravenous route pharmacokinetics, plasma protein binding, and uterine tissue dose metrics of bisphenol A: A physiologically based pharmacokinetic approach. *Toxicol Sci* 2005; 85: 823-838.

[46] Inoue H, Yuki G, Yokota H, et al. Bisphenol A glucuronidation and absorption in rat intestine. *Drug Metab Dispos* 2003; 31: 140-144.

[47] Yalcin EB, Kulkarni SR, Slitt AL, et al. Bisphenol A sulfonation is impaired in metabolic and liver disease. *Toxicol Appl Pharmacol* 2016; 292: 75-84.

[48] Krishnan K, Gagne M, Nong A, et al. Biomonitoring Equivalents for bisphenol A (BPA). *Regul Toxicol Pharmacol* 2010; 58: 18-24.

[49] González-Parra E, Herrero JA, Elewa U, et al. Bisphenol A in chronic kidney disease. *Int J Nephrol* 2013; 2013: 1-9.

[50] Kovacic P. How safe is bisphenol A? Fundamentals of toxicity: Metabolism, electron transfer and oxidative stress. *Med Hypotheses* 2010; 75: 1-4.

[51] INFOSAN. *BISFENOL A (BPA) – Estado actual de los conocimientos y medidas futuras de la OMS y la FAO*, https://www.who.int/foodsafety/fs_management/No_05_Bisphenol_A_Nov09_sp.pdf (2009, accessed 4 April 2019).

[52] Pottenger LH, Domoradzki JY, Markham DA, et al. The relative bioavailability and metabolism of bisphenol A in rats is dependent upon the route of administration. *Toxicol Sci* 2000; 54: 3-18.

[53] Volkel W, Bittner N, Dekant W. Detection of bisphenol A in human urine by LC-MS/MS. *Toxicol Appl Pharmacol* 2004; 197: 190.

[54] Doerge DR, Twaddle NC, Woodling KA, et al. Pharmacokinetics of bisphenol A in neonatal and adult rhesus monkeys. *Toxicol Appl Pharmacol* 2010; 248: 1-11.

[55] Taylor JA, vom Saal FS, Welshons W V., et al. Similarity of bisphenol A pharmacokinetics in rhesus monkeys and mice: Relevance for human exposure. *Environ Health Perspect* 2011; 119: 422-430.

[56] Centers for Disease Control and Prevention (CDC). National Center for Health Statistics (NCHS). NHANES Questionnaires, Datasets, and Related Documentation, https://wwwn.cdc.gov/nchs/nhanes/Default.aspx (accessed 24 February 2020).

[57] Park C, Choi W, Hwang M, et al. Associations between urinary phthalate metabolites and bisphenol A levels, and serum thyroid hormones among the Korean adult population - Korean National Environmental Health Survey (KoNEHS) 2012-2014. *Sci Total Environ* 2017; 584-585: 950-957.

[58] Bushnik T, Haines D, Levallois P, et al. Lead and bisphenol A concentrations in the Canadian population. *Heal reports* 2010; 21: 7-18.

[59] Hu J, Zhao H, Braun JM, et al. Associations of Trimester-Specific Exposure to Bisphenols with Size at Birth: A Chinese Prenatal Cohort Study. Environ Health Perspect 2019; 127: 107001.

[60] Morgan MK, Nash M, Barr DB, et al. Distribution, variability, and predictors of urinary bisphenol A levels in 50 North Carolina adults over a six-week monitoring period. *Environ Int* 2018; 112: 85-99.

[61] Cox KJ, Porucznik CA, Anderson DJ, et al. Exposure Classification and Temporal Variability in Urinary Bisphenol A Concentrations among Couples in Utah--The HOPE Study. *Environ Health Perspect* 2016; 124: 498-506.

[62] Park J-H, Hwang M-S, Ko A, et al. Risk assessment based on urinary bisphenol A levels in the general Korean population. *Environ Res* 2016; 150: 606-615.

[63] Derakhshan A, Shu H, Peeters RP, et al. Association of urinary bisphenols and triclosan with thyroid function during early pregnancy. *Environ Int* 2019; 133: 105123.

[64] Lewin A, Arbuckle TE, Fisher M, et al. Univariate predictors of maternal concentrations of environmental chemicals: The MIREC study. *Int J Hyg Environ Health* 2017; 220: 77-85.

[65] Aker AM, Ferguson KK, Rosario ZY, et al. The associations between prenatal exposure to triclocarban, phenols and parabens with gestational age and birth weight in northern Puerto Rico. *Environ Res* 2019; 169: 41-51.

[66] Dereumcaux C, Saoudi A, Pecheux M, et al. Biomarkers of exposure to environmental contaminants in French pregnant women from the Elfe cohort in 2011. *Environ Int* 2016; 97: 56-67.

[67] Kim JH, Hong Y-C. Increase of urinary malondialdehyde level by bisphenol A exposure: a longitudinal panel study. *Environ Health* 2017; 16: 8.

[68] Aung MT, Johns LE, Ferguson KK, et al. Thyroid hormone parameters during pregnancy in relation to urinary bisphenol A concentrations: A repeated measures study. *Environ Int* 2017; 104: 33-40.

[69] Philips EM, Jaddoe VW V, Asimakopoulos AG, et al. Bisphenol

and phthalate concentrations and its determinants among pregnant women in a population-based cohort in the Netherlands, 2004-5. *Environ Res* 2018; 161: 562-572.

[70] Ranciere F, Botton J, Slama R, et al. Exposure to Bisphenol A and Bisphenol S and Incident Type 2 Diabetes: A Case-Cohort Study in the French Cohort DESIR. *Environ Health Perspect* 2019; 127: 107013.

[71] Haug LS, Sakhi AK, Cequier E, et al. In-utero and childhood chemical exposome in six European mother-child cohorts. *Environ Int* 2018; 121: 751-763.

[72] Heffernan AL, Aylward LL, Toms LML, et al. Age-Related Trends in Urinary Excretion of Bisphenol A in Australian Children and Adults: Evidence from a Pooled Sample Study Using Samples of Convenience. *J Toxicol Environ Heal Part A* 2013; 76: 1039-1055.

[73] Youssef MM, El-Din EMS, Abu Shady MM, et al. Profile of urinary Bisphenol A (BPA) in association with age, sex and socio-economic standard in a sample of Egyptian children and adolescents. *Biosci Res* 2018; 15: 3404-3414.

[74] Christensen K, Lorber M. Exposure to BPA in Children—Media-Based and Biomonitoring-Based Approaches. *Toxics* 2014; 2: 134-157.

[75] LaKind JS, Pollock T, Naiman DQ, et al. Factors affecting interpretation of national biomonitoring data from multiple countries: BPA as a case study. *Environ Res* 2019; 173: 318-329.

[76] Amin MM, Ebrahim K, Hashemi M, et al. Association of exposure to Bisphenol A with obesity and cardiometabolic risk factors in children and adolescents. *Int J Environ Health Res* 2019; 29: 94-106.

[77] Song X, Miao M, Zhou X, et al. Bisphenol a exposure and sperm ache hydroxymethylation in men. *Int J Environ Res Public Health*; 16. Epub ahead of print 8 January 2019. DOI: 10.3390/ijerph16010152.

[78] Tian Y, Zhou X, Miao M, et al. Association of Bisphenol A Exposure with LINE-1 Hydroxymethylation in Human Semen. *Int J Environ Res Public Health*; 15. Epub ahead of print 17 August 2018. DOI: 10.3390/ijerph15081770.

[79] Hines CJ, Jackson M V, Deddens JA, et al. Urinary Bisphenol A (BPA) concentrations among workers in industries that manufacture and use BPA in the USA. *Ann Work Expo Heal* 2017; 61: 164-182.

[80] He Y, Miao M, Wu C, et al. Occupational Exposure Levels of Bisphenol A among Chinese Workers. *J Occup Health* 2009; 51: 432-436.

[81] Gerona RR, Pan J, Zota AR, et al. Direct measurement of Bisphenol A (BPA), BPA glucuronide and BPA sulfate in a diverse and low-income population of pregnant women reveals high exposure, with potential implications for previous exposure estimates: A cross-sectional study. *Environ Heal A Glob Access Sci Source* 2016; 15: 50.

[82] Vandentorren S, Zeman F, Morin L, et al. Bisphenol-A and phthalates contamination of urine samples by catheters in the Elfe pilot study: Implications for large-scale biomonitoring studies. *Environ Res* 2011; 111: 761-764.

[83] Huygh J, Clotman K, Malarvannan G, et al. Considerable exposure to the endocrine disrupting chemicals phthalates and bisphenol-A in intensive care unit (ICU) patients. *Environ Int* 2015; 81: 64-72.

[84] Wang F, Hua J, Chen M, et al. High urinary bisphenol A concentrations in workers and possible laboratory

abnormalities. *Occup Environ Med* 2012; 69: 679-684.

[85] Ndaw S, Remy AAA, Jargot DD, et al. Occupational exposure of cashiers to Bisphenol A via thermal paper: urinary biomonitoring study. *Int Arch Occup Environ Health* 2016; 89: 935-946.

[86] Mas S, Bosch-Panadero E, Abaigar P, et al. Influence of dialysis membrane composition on plasma bisphenol A levels during online hemodiafiltration. *PLoS One* 2018; 13: e0193288.

[87] Schoringhumer K, Cichna-Markl M. Sample clean-up with sol-gel enzyme and immunoaffinity columns for the determination of bisphenol A in human urine. *J Chromatogr B, Anal Technol Biomed life Sci* 2007; 850: 361-369.

[88] Shen Y, Liu T, Shi Y, et al. Bisphenol A analogs in patients with chronic kidney disease and dialysis therapy. *Ecotoxicol Environ Saf*; 185. Epub ahead of print 2019. DOI: 10.1016/j.ecoenv.2019.109684.

[89] Bosch-Panadero E, Mas S, Sanchez-Ospina D, et al. The Choice of Hemodialysis Membrane Affects Bisphenol A Levels in Blood. *J Am Soc Nephrol* 2016; 27: 1566-1574.

[90] Turgut F, Sungur S, Okur R, et al. Higher Serum Bisphenol A Levels in Diabetic Hemodialysis Patients. *BLOOD Purif* 2016; 42: 77-82.

[91] Quiroga B, Bosch RJ, Fiallos RA, et al. Online Hemodiafiltration Reduces Bisphenol A Levels. *Ther Apher Dial* 2017; 21: 96-101.

[92] Sajiki J, Hasegawa Y, Hashimoto H, et al. Determination of Bisphenol A (BPA) in Plasma of Hemodialysis Patients Using Three Methods: LC/ECD, LC/MS, and ELISA. *Toxicol Mech Methods* 2008; 18: 733-738.

[93] Murakami K, Ohashi A, Hori H, et al. Accumulation of bisphenol A in hemodialysis patients. *Blood Purif* 2007; 25: 290-294.

[94] Kanno Y, Okada H, Kobayashi T, et al. Effects of endocrine disrupting substance on estrogen receptor gene transcription in dialysis patients. *Ther Apher Dial* 2007; 11: 262-265.

[95] Liu X, Miao M, Zhou Z, et al. Exposure to bisphenol-A and reproductive hormones among male adults. *Environ Toxicol Pharmacol* 2015; 39: 934-941.

[96] Hines CJ, Jackson M V, Christianson AL, et al. Air, hand wipe, and surface wipe sampling for Bisphenol A (BPA) among workers in industries that manufacture and use BPA in the United States. *J Occup Environ Hyg* 2017; 14: 882-897.

[97] Xiao G, Wang R, Cai Y, et al. Effect of bisphenol A on semen quality of exposed workers: a pilot study. *Zhonghua Lao Dong Wei Sheng Zhi Ye Bing Za Zhi* 2009; 27: 741-743.

[98] Li D, Zhou Z, Qing D, et al. Occupational exposure to bisphenol-A (BPA) and the risk of self-reported male sexual dysfunction. *Hum Reprod* 2010; 25: 519-527.

[99] Li DK, Zhou Z, Miao M, et al. Relationship between urine bisphenol-A Level and declining male sexual function. *J Androl* 2010; 31: 500-506.

[100] Li D, Zhou ZZ, Miao MM, et al. Urine Bisphenol-a (BPA) Level in Relation to Semen Quality and Sexual Dysfunction. *EPIDEMIOLOGY* 2011; 95: 625-U616.

[101] Miao M, Zhou X, Li Y, et al. LINE-1 hypomethylation in spermatozoa is associated with Bisphenol A exposure. *Andrology* 2014; 2: 138-144.

[102] Miao M, Yuan W, Yang F, et al. Associations between Bisphenol A Exposure and Reproductive Hormones among Female Workers. *Int J Environ Res Public Health* 2015; 12: 13240-13250.

[103] Zhuang W, Wu K, Wang Y, et al. Association of Serum Bisphenol-A Concentration and Male Reproductive Function Among Exposed Workers. *Arch Environ Contam Toxicol* 2015; 68: 38-45.

[104] Heinälä M, Ylinen K, Tuomi T, et al. Assessment of Occupational Exposure to Bisphenol A in Five Different Production Companies in Finland. *Ann Work Expo Heal* 2017; 61: 44-55.

[105] Zhou Q, Miao M, Ran M, et al. Serum bisphenol-A concentration and sex hormone levels in men. *Fertil Steril* 2013; 100: 478-482.

[106] Kouidhi W, Thannimalay L, Soon CS, et al. Occupational exposure to bisphenol A (BPA) in a plastic injection molding factory in Malaysia. *Int J Occup Med Environ Health* 2017; 30: 743-750.

[107] Hanaoka T, Kawamura N, Hara K, et al. Urinary bisphenol A and plasma hormone concentrations in male workers exposed to bisphenol A diglycidyl ether and mixed organic solvents. *Occup Environ Med* 2002; 59: 625-628.

[108] He Y, Miao M, Herrinton LJ, et al. Bisphenol A levels in blood and urine in a Chinese population and the personal factors affecting the levels. *Environ Res* 2009; 109: 629-633.

[109] Waldman JM, Gavin Q, Anderson M, et al. Exposures to environmental phenols in Southern California firefighters and findings of elevated urinary benzophenone-3 levels. *Environ Int* 2016; 88: 281-287.

[110] Gonzalez N, Cunha SC, Monteiro C, et al. Quantification of eight bisphenol analogues in blood and urine samples of workers in a hazardous waste incinerator. *Environ Res* 2019; 176: 108576.

[111] Thayer KA, Taylor KW, Garantziotis S, et al. Bisphenol a, bisphenol s, and 4-hydro xyphenyl 4-isopro oxyphenyl sulfone (bpsip) in urine and blood of cashiers. *Environ Health Perspect* 2016; 124: 437-444.

[112] Hehn RS. NHANES Data Support Link between Handling of Thermal Paper Receipts and Increased Urinary Bisphenol A Excretion. *Environ Sci Technol* 2016; 50: 397-404.

[113] Motarjemi Y. *Encyclopedia of Food Safety*. First edit. Elsevier Inc. Epub ahead of print 2014. DOI: 10.5860/choice.52-0029.

[114] Tyl RW, Myers CB, Marr MC, et al. Two-generation reproductive toxicity study of dietary bisphenol A in CD-1 (Swiss) mice. *Toxicol Sci* 2008; 104: 362-384.

[115] Valentin J. Basic anatomical and physiological data for use in radiological protection: reference values. *Ann ICRP* 2002; 32: 1-277.

[116] Kurebayashi H, Nagatsuka S-I, Nemoto H, et al. Disposition of low doses of 14C-bisphenol A in male, female, pregnant, fetal, and neonatal rats. *Arch Toxicol* 2005; 79: 243-252.

[117] Völkel W, Bittner N, Dekant W, et al. Quantitation of bisphenol A and bisphenol A glucuronide in biological samples by high performance liquid chromatography-tandem mass spectrometry. *Drug Metab Dispos* 2005; 33: 1748-1757.

[118] Doerge DR, Twaddle NC, Vanlandingham M, et al. Pharmacokinetics of bisphenol A in neonatal and adult CD-1 mice: inter-species comparisons with

Sprague-Dawley rats and rhesus monkeys. *Toxicol Lett* 2011; 207: 298-305.

[119] Thayer KA, Doerge DR, Hunt D, et al. Pharmacokinetics of bisphenol A in humans following a single oral administration. *Environ Int* 2015; 83: 107-115.

[120] Russak EM, Bednarczyk EM. Impact of Deuterium Substitution on the Pharmacokinetics of Pharmaceuticals. *Annals of Pharmacotherapy* 2019; 53: 211-216.

[121] Schwabl P, Köppel S, Königshofer P, et al. Detection of Various Microplastics in Human Stool: A Prospective Case Series. *Ann Intern Med*. Epub ahead of print 2019. DOI: 10.7326/M19-0618.

[122] Vandenberg LN, Chahoud I, Heindel JJ, et al. Urinary, Circulating, and Tissue Biomonitoring Studies Indicate Widespread Exposure to Bisphenol A. *Environ Health Perspect* 2010; 118: 1055-1070.

[123] Stahlhut RW, Welshons W V., Swan SH. Bisphenol A data in NHANES suggest longer than expected half-life, substantial nonfood exposure, or both. *Environ Health Perspect* 2009; 117: 784-789.

[124] Vandenberg LN. Non-monotonic dose responses in studies of endocrine disrupting chemicals: Bisphenol a as a case study. *Dose-Response* 2014; 12: 259-276.

[125] Rochester JR. Bisphenol A and human health: A review of the literature. *Reprod Toxicol* 2013; 42: 132-155.

[126] Pjanic M. The role of polycarbonate monomer bisphenol-A in insulin resistance. *PeerJ*; 5. Epub ahead of print September 2017. DOI: 10.7717/peerj.3809.

[127] Angle BM, Do RP, Ponzi D, et al. Metabolic disruption in male mice due to fetal exposure to low but not high doses of bisphenol A (BPA): Evidence for effects on body weight, food intake, adipocytes, leptin, adiponectin, insulin and glucose regulation. *Reprod Toxicol* 2013; 42: 256-268.

Section 2

Coronavirus Disease 2019

Chapter 5

Consequences of COVID-19 Pandemic Including Endocrine and Metabolic Impacts

Hassan M. Heshmati

Abstract

A pandemic is an epidemic that spreads globally. Coronavirus disease 2019 (COVID-19) caused a major pandemic that affected human health and activities around the world since the beginning of 2020 and became a major international emergency. Through multiple paths, COVID-19 pandemic influenced life at individual, familial, societal, and environmental levels and led to a global economic recession. Severe acute respiratory syndrome coronavirus 2 (SARS-CoV-2) is the virus responsible for the disease. It invades the target cells by binding to angiotensin-converting enzyme 2 (ACE2). Endocrine and metabolic systems can be implicated in COVID-19 infection. Subjects with several comorbidities (e.g., hypertension, diabetes, and obesity) are more likely to be infected and are at a higher risk for complications and death from COVID-19. Wearing mask, social distancing, home confinement, and isolation have been recommended and implemented in several countries to curb the spread of the outbreak. Vaccination remains the best protective measure. Different vaccines are now available and have been used. The worldwide impact of COVID-19 pandemic may last several years.

Keywords: pandemic, COVID-19, consequences, endocrine and metabolic systems

1. Introduction

A pandemic is an epidemic that spreads globally, crosses international boundaries, and affects large number of people (**Figure 1**) [1, 2].

Through multiple mechanisms (e.g., infection and confinement/isolation), pandemics can influence life at individual, familial, societal, and environmental levels [3].

COVID-19 pandemic became a global health and economic crisis of the 21st century, representing one of the most profound medical, societal, and economic challenges in modern times [4–7]. Endocrine and metabolic systems can be involved in COVID-19 infection [8–48]. Diabetes and obesity negatively impact immune system and increase the risk of infection and morbidity/mortality due to COVID-19 [8–12, 14, 23–25, 31, 33–37].

Multiple COVID-19 vaccines are now available and have been used worldwide [49–53].

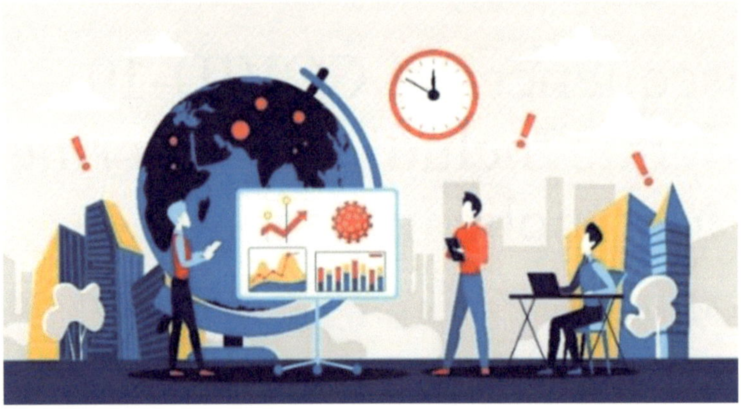

Figure 1.
Pandemics affect large number of people in multiple countries.

2. Pandemics

2.1 History of pandemics

Numerous pandemics have occurred throughout the history of mankind, the most recent being the COVID-19 pandemic [1, 2, 4–6].

Important pandemics that occurred over the last 1,500 years are reported in **Table 1** (non-exhaustive list). The deadliest pandemics were the Plague of Justinian, the Black Death, and the Spanish Flu.

Pandemic Name	Pathogen	Vector	Date	Mortality
Plague of Justinian	Yersinia pestis	Fleas	541–750	Up to 100,000,000
Black Death	Yersinia pestis	Fleas	1347–1351	Up to 200,000,000
Spanish Flu	H1N1 virus	Avian	1918–1919	Up to 100,000,000
Asian Flu	H2N2 virus	Avian	1957–1958	Up to 4,000,000
Hong Kong Flu	H3N2 virus	Avian	1968–1969	Up to 4,000,000
Swine Flu	H1N1 virus	Pigs	2009–2010	Up to 250,000
COVID-19	SARS-CoV-2	Unknown	2019-present	At least 4,362,000*

**As of August 17, 2021.*

Table 1.
Important pandemics over the last 1,500 years (non-exhaustive list).

2.2 Consequences of pandemics

Through multiple paths (e.g., infection and confinement/isolation), pandemics can influence life at individual, familial, societal, and environmental levels [3].

At the individual level, there are health consequences (e.g., infection caused by the pathogen, metabolic diseases, mental disorders, impact on pre-existing conditions, and eventually death), financial challenges (mainly due to unemployment), and educational consequences (due to remote learning).

At the familial level, the prolonged presence of parents and children at home can promote domestic violence.

At the societal level, the limitation of social life and activities will have major economic consequences for several businesses (e.g., agriculture, restaurant, hotel, store, airline, cruise, convention, concert, sport event, museum, movie, and theater).

At the environmental level, the confinement may have some health benefits, at least for short term, due to a reduction in air pollution mainly secondary to the decrease in circulating cars and flying planes. This can also positively impact the life of animals and plants.

3. COVID-19 pandemic

3.1 Virus

In January 2020, Chinese authorities announced the isolation of a new type of coronavirus, SARS-CoV-2, following the occurrence in December 2019 of several pneumonia cases of unknown etiology. On March 11, 2020, the World Health Organization (WHO) declared COVID-19 a pandemic.

COVID-19 is caused by one of the coronaviruses in the family of Coronaviridae. The virus belongs to genera Betacoronavirus and is the seventh coronavirus known to cause human diseases. It is a spherical or pleomorphic enveloped, non-segmented, single-stranded, positive-sense RNA virus. The genome of the virus is composed of 29,903 nucleotides. The virus is made up of four main structural proteins: spike (S), membrane (M), envelope (E), and nucleocapsid (N) proteins (**Figure 2**) [4–6, 14, 25, 29, 38, 54, 55].

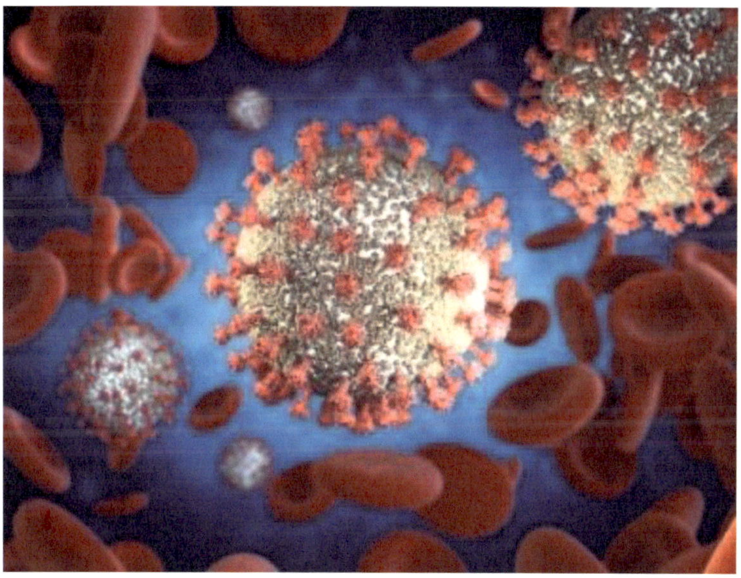

Figure 2.
SARS-CoV-2.

SARS-CoV-2 evolves over time and like other viruses is subject to mutations. The mutated virus is referred to as a variant of the original virus. Several variants of SARS-CoV-2 have been reported (e.g., Alpha, Beta, Delta, Epsilon, Eta, Gamma, Iota, Kappa, Lambda, Theta, and Zeta). They were initially detected in countries like the United Kingdom (UK), South Africa, Brazil, and India. Some variants are more transmissible and aggressive and may be more resistant to the current vaccines. The Delta variant has created serious concerns in several countries, especially in the USA where it became the dominant variant affecting adults, adolescents, and children, and causing spike in hospitalizations.

3.2 COVID-19 origin, mode of transmission, and action

The exact origin of SARS-CoV-2 has been subject of multiple debates and speculations (bats to humans through Huanan Seafood Market or release from a research laboratory, in Wuhan, Hubei Province, China). According to the former director of Centers for Disease Control and Prevention in the United States of America (USA), the virus most likely originated from the Wuhan research laboratory. The accidental or intentional release of the virus remains to be established.

Human-to-human transmission occurs mainly by direct contact or by droplets spread by infected subjects through cough or sneeze. The virus can survive in the environment from a few hours to a few days, depending on the conditions. The nose, mouth, and ocular mucosa are the major way of transmission (**Figure 3**).

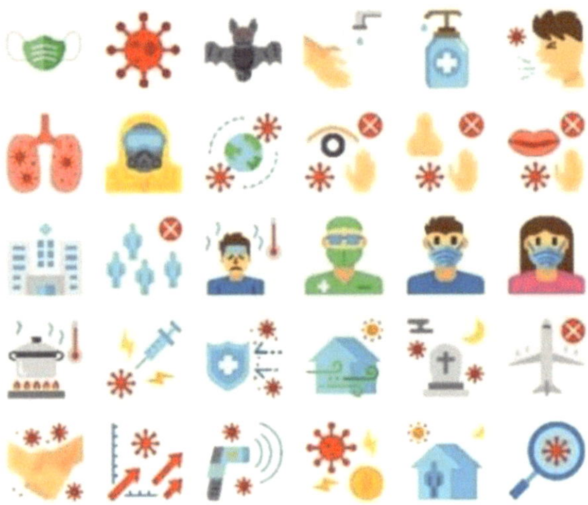

Figure 3.
Mode of transmission of SARS-CoV-2.

The virus uses the host cell membrane protein receptors to enter and infect the cell. The most well-described cell membrane protein receptor is ACE2 (a zinc metalloprotease). First, the virus spike protein binds to ACE2. Then, there is an internalization of ACE2 with a subsequent reduction of cell surface ACE2 enzymatic activity [14, 25, 29, 38, 55]. ACE2 is expressed in several organs including endocrine glands. It is abundant in the epithelia of the lung and intestine. Infected cells undergo apoptosis or necrosis and trigger inflammatory responses.

3.3 COVID-19 diagnostic tests

The Food and Drug Administration in the USA has approved two tests for diagnosing COVID-19 infection. The antigen test detects certain proteins in the virus. The polymerase chain reaction test detects genetic material of the virus. For both tests, the fluid sample is collected using a nasal swab (**Figure 4**).

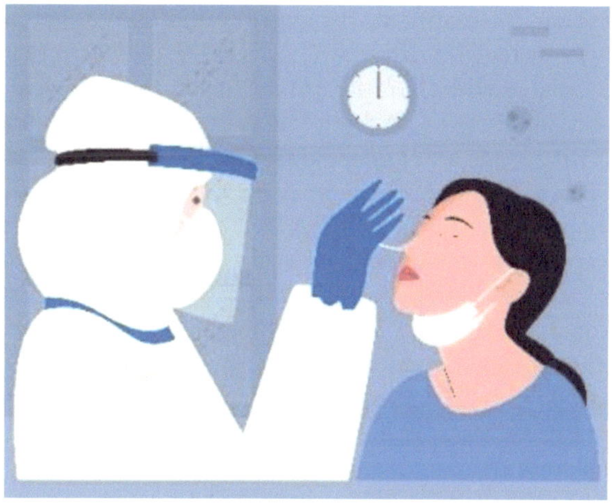

Figure 4.
COVID-19 diagnostic tests use a nasal swab to collect fluid sample.

3.4 COVID-19 consequences

Through infection and confinement/isolation, COVID-19 can influence life at individual, familial, societal, and environmental levels (**Figure 5**) [3].

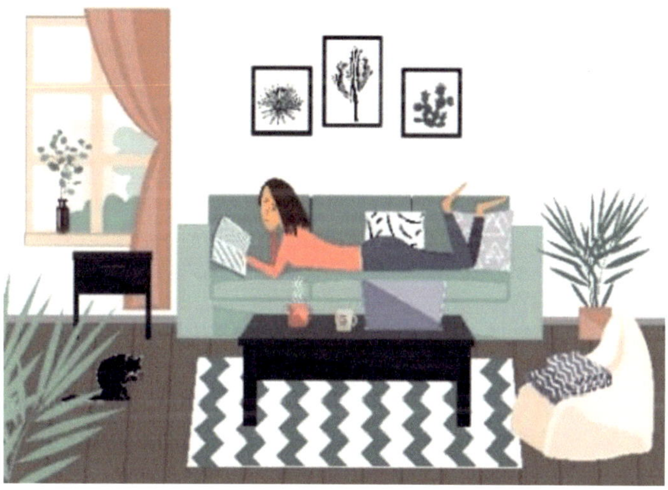

Figure 5.
COVID-19 pandemic led to confinement/isolation.

3.4.1 Individual

3.4.1.1 Health consequences

3.4.1.1.1 Global health

COVID-19 has placed a significant burden upon healthcare worldwide. COVID-19 can target different systems that express ACE2 (respiratory, cardiovascular, neurological, gastrointestinal, endocrine, others). Although lung has been reported to be one of the most affected organs, the contribution of intestinal involvement to the clinical course of the disease and its treatment (through gut microbiota) has been highly speculated [54]. All age groups may be affected. The disease is more severe in men [11, 12].

COVID-19 is associated with alterations in the host immunological status including an increase in pro-inflammatory cytokines. The surge of pro-inflammatory factors ("cytokine storm") may cause host organ damage such as lung damage resulting in severe respiratory failure [8, 38]. Subjects infected with COVID-19 can be asymptomatic, have mild symptoms recovering within 1 to 2 weeks, or be severely affected (e.g., severe pneumonia and cardiogenic shock) with the ultimate risk of death. Common symptoms include fever, dry cough, dyspnea, arthralgia, myalgia, ageusia (loss of taste), and anosmia (loss of smell). COVID-19 symptoms can sometimes last several months. The damage to the lungs, heart, and brain can increase the risk of long-term symptoms (long haulers). Older subjects (> 65 years), black subjects, smokers, and subjects with immunodeficiency, cardiac and respiratory diseases, cancer, hypertension, diabetes, obesity, and dyslipidemia are considered high-risk populations [8–12, 14, 23–25, 31, 33–37, 39]. Among COVID-19 mortality cases in Wuhan, China, the main associated comorbidities were hypertension (54%), diabetes (42%), and cardiac disease (19%) [9].

The public health recommendations during the COVID-19 pandemic resulted in social distancing and home confinement/isolation. More than 4 billion people worldwide have experienced the COVID-19 mobility restriction. The life in home confinement and self-isolation for a long period has significant negative health consequences due to alterations in lifestyle (eating behavior and physical activity) and mental status, and the impact on pre-existing diseases [3, 21, 22, 31, 32, 40, 42, 56–58].

The changes in lifestyle (e.g., unhealthy diet and reduced physical activity) which affect both adults and children, can lead to weight gain (overweight or obesity). Sedentarism can cause a very rapid loss of muscle mass (up to 10% after 30 days) with degenerative changes of the neuromuscular system and reduced cardiorespiratory fitness [21]. The confinement and isolation, especially if associated with unemployment and financial challenges, can negatively influence psychological health, and promote anxiety and depression, especially in women [3, 40, 57, 58]. It may also impact access to health care (e.g., medications, physicians, and hospital beds) for the management of pre-existing medical conditions (e.g., heart disease, cancer, and diabetes) [3].

Death can result from direct consequences of the viral infection, mental complications of confinement/isolation with the risk of suicide, or aggravation of pre-existing diseases (**Figure 6**).

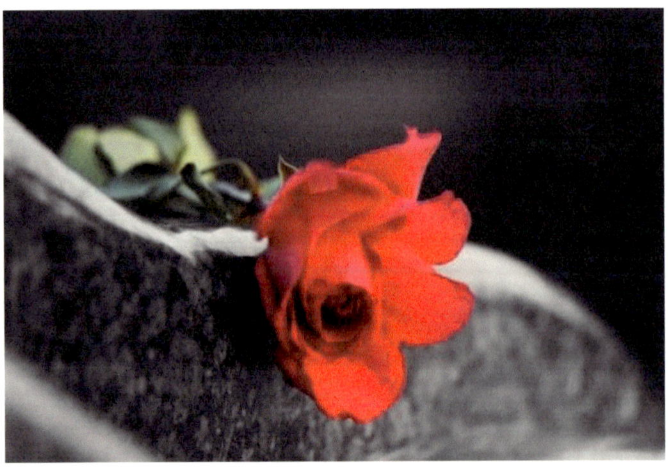

Figure 6.
Death from COVID-19 pandemic affected millions of people worldwide.

The extent of death from COVID-19 pandemic as of August 17, 2021 is reported in **Table 2**. African countries had a low mortality rate, at least at the beginning of the pandemic, that can be explained in part by the existence of less indoor activities (less exposure to the virus) and younger population.

Country	Total Population	Infected Subject	Mortality
World	**Around 7,900,000,000**	**At least 207,173,000**	**At least 4,362,000**
USA	Around 333,000,000	At least 36,385,000	At least 615,000
Brazil	Around 214,000,000	At least 20,350,000	At least 568,000
India	Around 1,395,000,000	At least 32,225,000	At least 431,000
Mexico	Around 130,000,000	At least 3,091,000	At least 248,000
Peru	Around 33,000,000	At least 2,132,000	At least 197,000
Russia	Around 146,000,000	At least 6,621,000	At least 171,000
UK	Around 68,000,000	At least 6,267,000	At least 130,000
Italy	Around 60,000,000	At least 4,440,000	At least 128,000
Colombia	Around 51,000,000	At least 4,864,000	At least 123,000
Indonesia	Around 277,000,000	At least 3,871,000	At least 118,000
France	Around 65,000,000	At least 6,311,000	At least 111,000
Argentina	Around 46,000,000	At least 5,080,000	At least 108,000

Table 2.
Extent of infection and death from COVID-19 pandemic in 12 countries ranked by descending order of death (WHO data, as of August 17, 2021).

Between March and October 2020, COVID-19 became the third leading cause of death in the USA (after heart disease and cancer) for persons aged 45 to 84 years [7].

For several months and mainly due to political reasons, the magnitude and gravity of COVID-19 pandemic were not taken seriously in the USA at federal and some state levels. According to the former COVID-19 task force coordinator, with an appropriate management and policy, hundreds of thousands of lives could have been saved.

3.4.1.1.2 Endocrine and metabolic systems

Several endocrine and metabolic systems can be impacted by COVID-19 infection (**Figure 7**) [8–48]. Findings in this area are evolving and long-term effects of COVID-19 infection remain unknown.

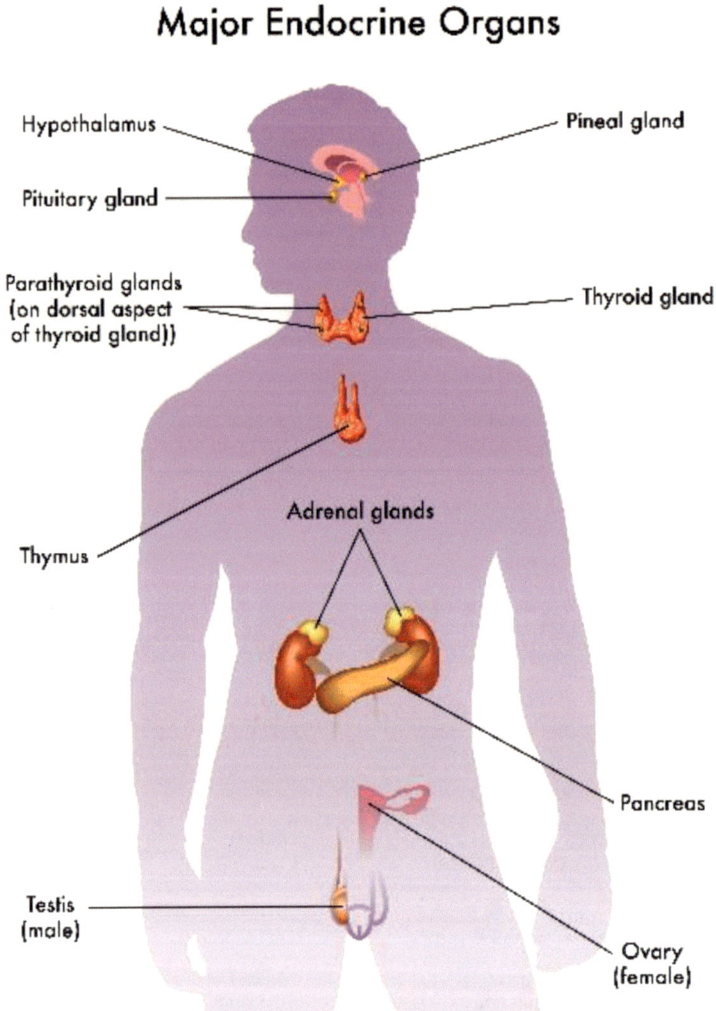

Figure 7.
Different endocrine systems can be impacted by COVID-19 infection.

3.4.1.1.2.1 Hypothalamus, pituitary

The hypothalamus and pituitary tissues do express ACE2 and can theoretically be targeted by SARS-CoV-2. However, there are no solid data on hypothalamic–pituitary dysfunction in subjects affected by COVID-19 [8, 10, 12, 14].

In subjects with treated diabetes insipidus, the priority should be to avoid hyponatremia [8].

Management of pituitary tumors without signs of emergency (e.g., visual deterioration and apoplexy) can be differed for several months [16].

3.4.1.1.2.2 Thyroid

ACE2 receptors have been located in the thyroid. Data on thyroid involvement during COVID-19 infection are relatively limited [8, 10, 12, 14, 17, 18].

In severe cases of COVID-19, subjects may present with nonthyroidal illness syndrome [17]. Several cases of onset of subacute thyroiditis have been reported in subjects with COVID-19 infection [12, 14]. COVID-19 can be a precipitating factor for the initiation or relapse of Graves' disease [8, 10]. In subjects receiving antithyroid drugs, because symptoms of agranulocytosis (a rare side effect of antithyroid drugs) can overlap with COVID-19, special attention is needed [12].

Diagnostic procedures and surgery for thyroid nodules can be postponed in most cases [8, 30]. The timing of surgery should be carefully decided for subjects with thyroid cancer [19, 30].

3.4.1.1.2.3 Parathyroid

Data on parathyroid disorders and COVID-19 infection are relatively rare. In case of hyperparathyroidism, surgery can be postponed without major clinical impact [20].

3.4.1.1.2.4 Adrenal

ACE2 is expressed in the adrenal gland. Impaired adrenocortical response has been reported in subjects with COVID-19 infection consistent with central adrenal insufficiency [15].

Subjects with Cushing's disease or syndrome may be at higher risk of COVID-19 infection since excess cortisol production has immunosuppressive effect [8, 12]. Medical treatment is recommended as first-line therapy for most of these subjects during the COVID-19 pandemic.

Adrenal insufficiency may create a potentially increased risk of acquiring COVID-19 infection as this condition is associated with impaired immunity. Subjects with adrenal insufficiency may be at higher risk of medical complications and increased mortality in case of COVID-19 infection. If COVID-19 infection is suspected in subjects with adrenal insufficiency, a prompt increase in dose of the replacement therapy is indicated to avoid adrenal crisis [8, 10, 12–14]. Subjects with known adrenal insufficiency and COVID-19 may require parenteral glucocorticoid treatment with careful monitoring of serum potassium [12, 13].

3.4.1.1.2.5 Pancreas

ACE2 is expressed in pancreas (both exocrine and endocrine pancreas). Physical inactivity leads to insulin resistance and systemic inflammation with subsequent metabolic consequences [21, 22]. COVID-19 infection, through multiple mechanisms, may impair the function of the endocrine pancreas and promote or aggravate diabetes [10, 14, 23].

Chronic hyperglycemia in subjects with diabetes negatively impacts immune system and increases the risk of infection and morbidity/mortality due to COVID-19 (**Figure 8**) [8–12, 14, 23–25]. It is important to maintain a good glycemic control in subjects with diabetes to reduce the risk of COVID-19 infection. In case of COVID-19 infection, the outpatient plasma glucose goal is 72–144 mg/dL with a hemoglobin A1c goal less than 7%. Plasma glucose should be monitored at least twice a day. Insulin is the preferred treatment in hospitalized subjects with the use of continuous glucose monitoring [12].

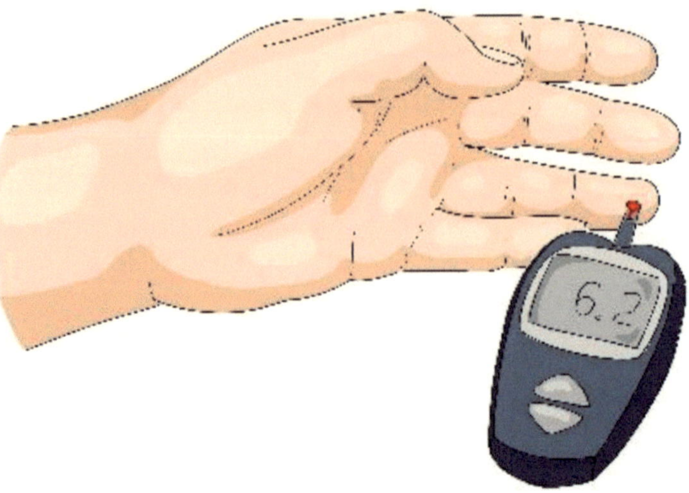

Figure 8.
COVID-19 pandemic can promote diabetes or be aggravated by diabetes.

3.4.1.1.2.6 Testis

There is a high level of ACE2 expression in the testis (e.g., Sertoli cells, Leydig cells, and spermatogonia). COVID-19 infection may cause Sertoli cells, Leydig cells, and seminiferous tubules damages resulting in low serum testosterone levels and altered sperm quality [10, 12, 14, 26–28].

Men with COVID-19 are exposed to worse outcome than women, possibly due to sex differences in immune response [11, 12].

3.4.1.1.2.7 Ovary

ACE2 is expressed in the ovary. However, data on ovarian function and COVID-19 infection are limited [12, 14]. COVID-19 infection may disturb the female reproductive system and cause menstrual disorder, infertility, and fetal distress [29].

3.4.1.1.2.8 Adipose tissue

Adipose tissue expresses ACE2. The unhealthy diet and reduced physical activity promoted by confinement can lead to overweight or obesity, especially in high-income countries/families [31, 32]. Low-income countries/families are exposed to food insecurity, malnutrition, and weight loss [31].

With higher adipose tissue mass, more receptors (ACE2) would be available for SARS-CoV-2, exposing subjects to COVID-19 [10]. Subjects with overweight/obesity may experience a more serious COVID-19 infection through several mechanisms (e.g., inflammation, impaired immunity, mechanical lung dysfunction, impact of comorbidities, and vitamin D deficiency) (**Figure 9**) [8–11, 14, 31, 33–37]. These subjects require weight reduction using the appropriate tools as indicated (e.g., diet, exercise, drug, medical device, and bariatric surgery) [36, 37, 59–62]. All precautions should be taken to avoid infection. Subjects with obesity and COVID-19 who require treatment in intensive care units present challenges in their management (e.g., difficulty for moving, for intubating, and for obtaining diagnostic imaging) [8].

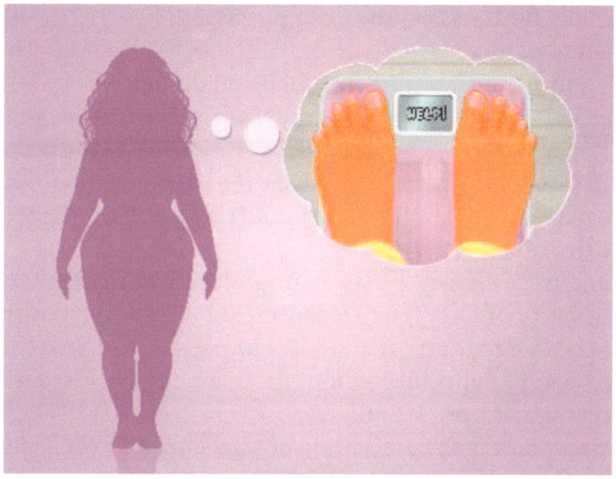

Figure 9.
COVID-19 pandemic can promote overweight/obesity or be aggravated by overweight/obesity.

3.4.1.1.2.9 Lipids

The "cytokine storm" caused by COVID-19 produces an immune-mediated inflammatory dyslipidemia (e.g., decreased high-density lipoprotein cholesterol and low-density lipoprotein cholesterol, increased triglycerides, and increased lipoprotein oxidation) [38].

Dyslipidemia is one of the most common comorbidities in the general population and in subjects with COVID-19. It can potentially increase the severity and mortality of COVID-19. This increased risk is more pronounced with older age, male gender, and presence of hypertension [39].

3.4.1.1.2.10 Nutrition (calories, macronutrients, electrolytes, vitamins) and exercise

During COVID-19 confinement, a healthy lifestyle is essential (**Figure 10**). An optimal nutrition (e.g., calories, macronutrients, electrolytes, and vitamins) is

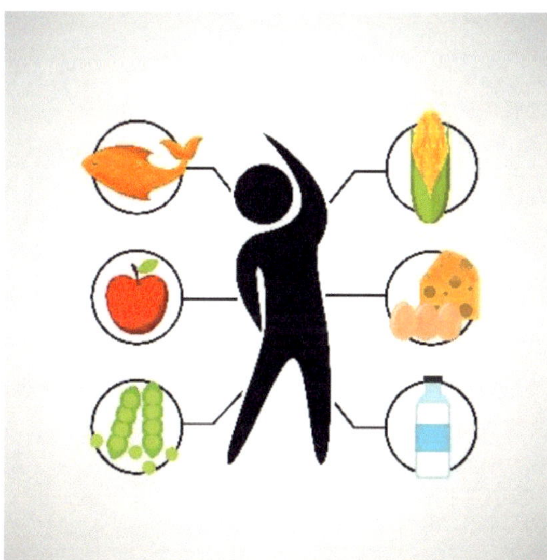

Figure 10.
Healthy lifestyle is essential during COVID-19 pandemic.

important, especially for boosting the immune system [21, 31, 33, 40–44, 47, 48]. It is recommended to reduce the daily energy intake by 15–25% with more energy during breakfast and less energy during lunch and dinner.

Diet should be balanced and contain fruits, vegetables, whole grains, low-fat dairy products, and olive oil, with adequate hydration. The consumption of sugar, saturated fat, and salt should be reduced. COVID-19 infected-subjects, especially those who are hospitalized, are at risk of malnutrition and need adequate nutritional support [8].

Electrolytes and trace elements play an important role in the management of COVID-19. The severity of COVID-19 is associated with lower serum concentrations of sodium, potassium, and calcium. It is important to assess the levels of electrolytes and trace elements throughout the course of the disease to establish appropriate corrective actions [45, 46].

Vitamins are important in the prevention of viral infection. Subjects at risk of or with respiratory viral infection should receive vitamin C and vitamin D. Particular attention should be paid to the treatment of subjects with hypovitaminosis D [8, 11, 12].

Safe handling of food, from production to consumption, is critical to reduce the risk of viral dissemination.

Daily exercise (e.g., low to medium-intensity exercise) is essential for preventing the negative impact of inactivity and improving health [21, 40].

COVID-19 has caused a major disruption in the management of subjects with endocrine and metabolic disorders. The services offered by healthcare systems must adapt rapidly. Outpatient management with remote advice and support services need to be organized [23, 30]. Routine in-person appointments are not recommended in order to avoid crowds in waiting rooms [9]. Elective surgical procedures should be postponed when possible.

3.4.1.2 Financial consequences

Unemployment may cause financial challenges at the individual level and this can affect both physical and mental health (**Figure 11**) [31, 40]. Between February and May 2020, the number of unemployed Americans rose by more than 14 million.

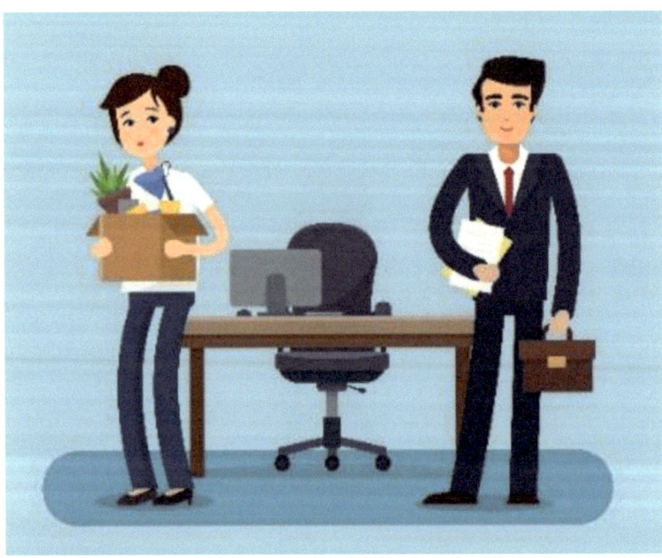

Figure 11.
Unemployment caused by COVID-19 pandemic may lead to individual financial challenges.

3.4.1.3 Educational consequences

For the current generation of young people (children and adolescents), the disrupted education due to remote learning and lack of in-person classes during an extensive period of confinement and social distancing can negatively impact the quality of education and social skills (**Figure 12**).

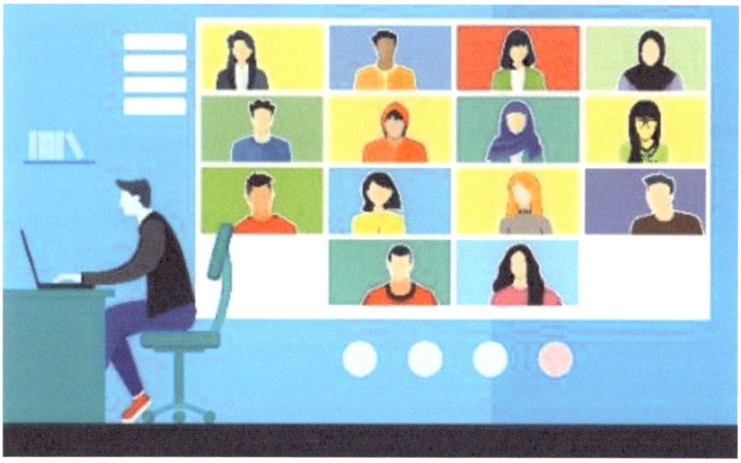

Figure 12.
The switch to remote learning during COVID-19 pandemic may impact the quality of education and social skills of the current generation of students.

3.4.2 Familial

During the enforced COVID-19 home confinement, there is an important decrease in the amount of familial/social activities (e.g., interactions with other individuals and entertainment), associated with a lower life satisfaction [63].

Confinement, isolation, and prolonged presence of parents and children expose to the risk of domestic violence. Children and their mothers are particularly vulnerable (**Figure 13**) [64].

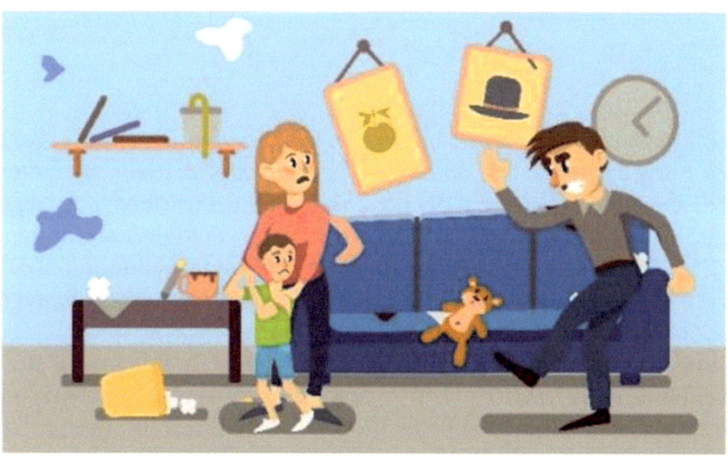

Figure 13.
The confinement following COVID-19 pandemic can promote domestic violence.

3.4.3 Societal

COVID-19 pandemic led to a global economic recession [40]. According to a report released by the World Bank, in 2020, the world economy probably shrank by 4.3% (equivalent of $3.9 trillion).

The financial burden of COVID-19 is mainly due to confinement and limitation of social life. These restrictions lead to the limitation or closing of several businesses (with the subsequent increase of unemployment) affecting the income from agriculture, restaurant, hotel, store, airline, cruise, convention, concert, sport event, museum, movie, and theater (non-exhaustive list) and causing health issues, all contributing to a decrease in productivity and an increase in national debt.

Reducing social inequalities should become a priority for all countries to build resilience during the pandemic.

The pandemic also impacted medical research for hospitals and pharmaceutical companies by creating limitations in implementation and conduct of clinical trials in different countries, especially when in-person visits are necessary.

3.4.4 Environmental

The lockdown measures of COVID-19 pandemic caused a temporary reduction in global air pollution secondary to the decrease of anthropogenic activities (e.g., less circulating cars and flying planes) (**Figure 14**) [65–67].

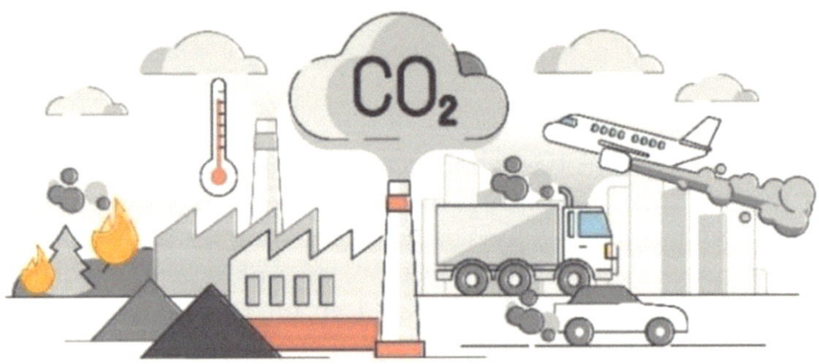

Figure 14.
The confinement due to COVID-19 pandemic temporarily reduced air pollution by decreasing the anthropogenic activities.

Most polluted cities are located in Asia, especially in India, China, and Pakistan. Results of a study using satellite observations at the continental scale from January to May 2020 showed a substantial decrease in the concentrations of nitrogen dioxide (maximum reduction of 33% in East Asia), sulfur dioxide (maximum reduction of 41% in East Asia), and aerosol optical depth (maximum reduction of 37% in South Asia) during the lockdown period of 2020 compared to their averages for the baseline period (2015–2019) over all continents [65].

According to WHO, ambient air pollution was responsible for 4.2 million deaths worldwide in 2016 (mainly from respiratory infection, chronic obstructive ulmonary disease, ischemic heart disease, stroke, and lung cancer).
Any reduction in global air pollution, even for a short period of time, may

theoretically have some health and financial benefits for humans. It can also be beneficial for animals and plants.

3.5 COVID-19 prevention

3.5.1 General precautions

In many locations affected by COVID-19 infection, wearing mask, social distancing, and lockdown (with the possibility to work from home) became mandatory to prevent the expansion of the disease in the general population and the subsequent medical challenges for the healthcare system (**Figure 15**). In addition, subjects were encouraged to wear gloves when appropriate and do careful hand washing, especially before eating and drinking.

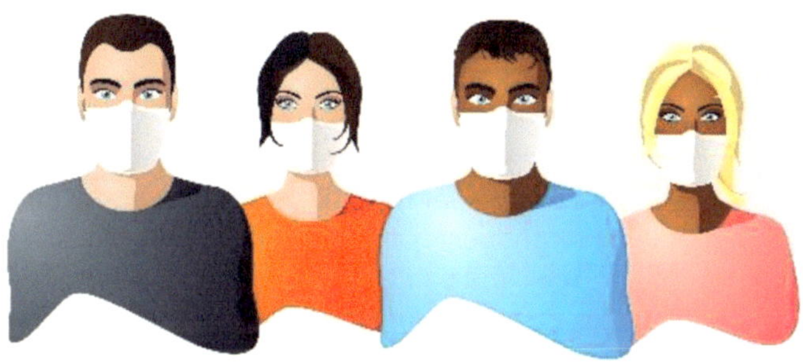

Figure 15.
Wearing mask is a simple but very efficient way to protect against COVID-19 infection.

Politicization of wearing mask in some countries (e.g., USA) created medical challenges in the control of the pandemic.

3.5.2 Vaccination

Vaccination is the cheapest and most effective way to protect against COVID-19 infection. Vaccine development is a lengthy process that usually takes 10–15 years, but development of COVID-19 vaccines followed a very fast pace mainly due to collaborative efforts of research institutions and active engagement of regulatory agencies.

Several vaccine candidates have been investigated by various companies in different countries using multiple vaccine platforms (e.g., live-attenuated, inactivated, protein subunit, virus-like particle, replicating viral vector, non-replicating viral vector, DNA, and mRNA) [49–53]. Several vaccines were designed to use the SARS-CoV-2 spike protein or part of it as the immunogen. As of August 17, 2021, 21 COVID-19 vaccines have been approved or authorized for emergency use by at least 1 country. In the USA, Pfizer/BioNTech vaccine was first authorized for emergency use in subjects aged 16 years and older and later for adolescents aged 12 to 15 years. A partial list of the approved/authorized vaccines is reported in **Table 3**. Several clinical trials of additional COVID-19 vaccines are currently ongoing (44 trials in Phase 1, 59 trials in Phase 2, and 29 trials in Phase 3).

Company	Type of Vaccine	Number of Country Approval/Authorization
Oxford/AstraZeneca (UK)	Non-replicating viral vector	121
Pfizer/BioNTech (USA/Germany)	mRNA	97
Gamaleya (1) (Russia)	Non-replicating viral vector	71
Moderna (USA)	mRNA	68
Sinopharm Beijing (China)	Inactivated	60
Janssen (USA)	Non-replicating viral vector	59
Serum Institute of India (India)	Non-replicating viral vector	45
Sinovac (China)	Inactivated	39
Gamaleya (2) (Russia)	Non-replicating viral vector	12
Bharat Biotech (India)	Inactivated	9
CanSino (China)	Non-replicating viral vector	8

Table 3.
Top 11 COVID-19 vaccines approved/authorized by at least 1 country ranked by descending order of number of country approval/authorization (as of August 17, 2021).

As of August 17, 2021, the number of COVID-19 vaccine doses administered was more than 4,452,000,000. In most locations, the vaccination prioritized the healthcare workers, old subjects, and subjects with comorbidities. The mRNA vaccines need to be stored and transported at very low temperatures. This requirement may prevent effective distribution of these vaccines to areas with limited availability of specialized freezers. Viral spread will continue to cause significant health and economic issues until a sufficient number of subjects are vaccinated and herd immunity is achieved (**Figure 16**).

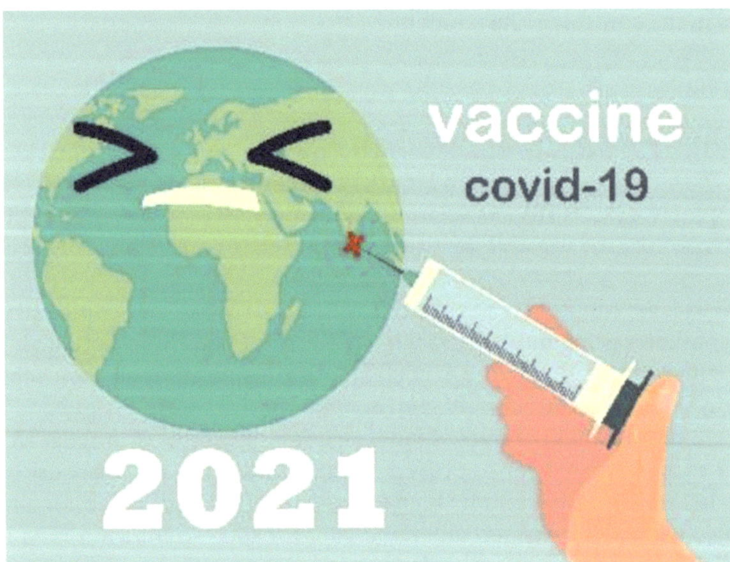

Figure 16.
There is a need to vaccinate a minimum number of subjects worldwide against COVID-19 to reach herd immunity.

COVID-19 vaccines have a high efficacy (up to 95%) by providing significant protection against severe disease, hospitalization, and death. The duration of immunity after the first full vaccination is unknown. COVID-19 vaccine boosters are most likely necessary for all vaccinated subjects. In the USA, very recently, Pfizer/BioNTech and Moderna received authorization for an extra dose of vaccine in immunocompromised subjects. Some of the currently available vaccines provide partial to complete protection against SARS-CoV-2 variants.

COVID-19 vaccines are overall safe and well tolerated. Subjects may develop minor side effects (e.g., swelling, redness, and pain at injection site, fever, headache, tiredness, muscle pain, chills, and nausea) lasting usually 1 or 2 days after the injection. In rare cases, subjects may develop anaphylaxis, myocarditis/pericarditis, and thrombosis. Long-term side effects of COVID-19 vaccines are currently unknown. Limited data are available regarding vaccine safety in pregnancy.

There are a significant number of subjects with vaccine hesitancy for a variety of reasons including concerns about the unknown or undisclosed side effects of the vaccines, absence of full vaccine approval, ignorance, misinformation, selfishness, and political influence (mainly in the USA).

3.6 COVID-19 treatment

The standard management of COVID-19 infection is based on supportive treatment with lung-protective ventilation and dexamethasone. Several drugs have also been investigated and used for the treatment of COVID-19 infection. They include antiviral agents (e.g., remdesivir) and monoclonal antibodies (e.g., casirivimab + imdevimab and sotrovimab) (**Figure 17**) [68].

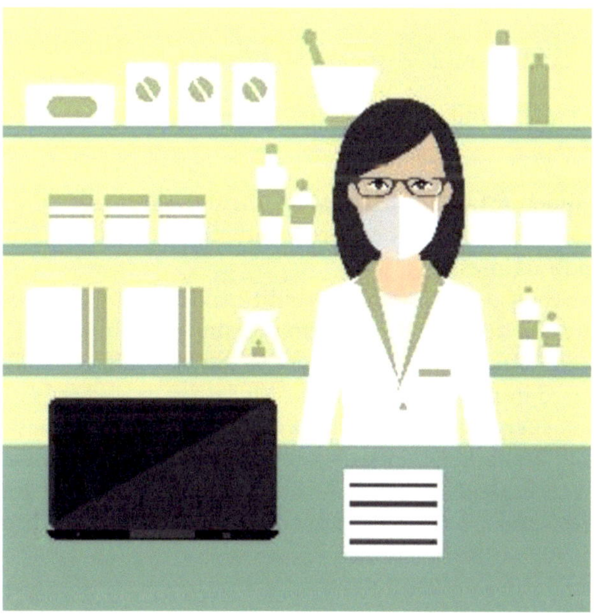

Figure 17.
Several drugs to treat COVID-19 infection are currently used or under investigation.

4. Life with COVID-19 pandemic

The COVID-19 pandemic may last several years and can cause dramatic changes in society, affecting our lives for generations to come. The precautions necessary to avoid infection or transmission of the virus may stay in effect for a long period. This has significant impact on life at different levels (e.g., family, profession, gathering, traveling, hand shaking, hugging, kissing, and love making). The new normal, even at a very personal level, may be very different and somehow odd (**Figure 18**).

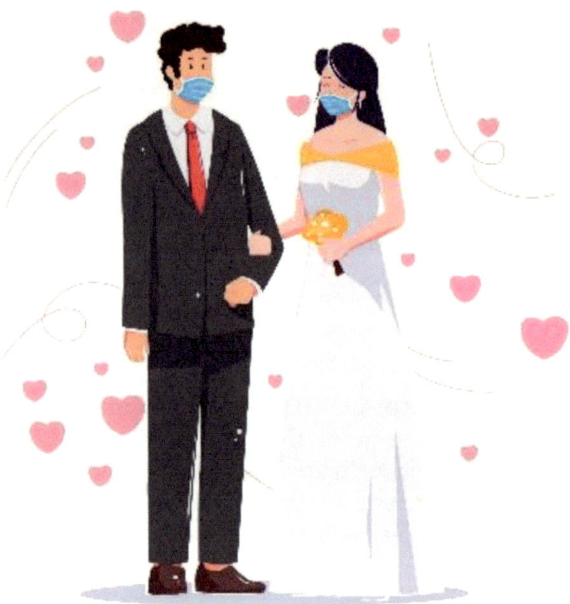

Figure 18.
The new normal after COVID-19 pandemic may look odd but necessary.

5. Conclusions

COVID-19 pandemic became a global health and economic crisis of the 21st century. It represents one of the most profound medical, societal, and economic challenges in modern times.

The pandemic caused substantial morbidity and mortality. Almost all organs and biological systems are directly or indirectly impacted by COVID-19. The presence of diabetes and obesity contributes to a worse prognosis of COVID-19 infection due to impaired immune function.

Wearing mask, social distancing, home confinement, and isolation have been recommended and implemented in most countries to curb the spread of the outbreak. Mass quarantine leads to major health and social consequences.

Several efficient and safe vaccines are now available and have been used worldwide.

Conflict of interest

The author declares no conflict of interest.

Author details

Hassan M. Heshmati
Endocrinology Metabolism Consulting, LLC, Anthem, AZ, USA

*Address all correspondence to: hassanheshmati@yahoo.com

References

[1] Samal J. A historical exploration of pandemics of some selected diseases in the world. International Journal of Health Sciences and Research. 2014;**4**:165-169.

[2] Piret J, Boivin G. Pandemics throughout history. Frontiers in Microbiology. 2021;**11**:631736. DOI: 10.3389/fmicb.2020.631736

[3] Yen-Hao Chu I, Alam P, Larson HJ, Lin L. Social consequences of mass quarantine during epidemics: A systematic review with implications for the COVID-19 response. Journal of Travel Medicine. 2020;**27**:1-14. DOI: 10.1093/jtm/taaa192

[4] Sahin AR, Erdogan A, Mutlu Agaoglu P, et al. 2019 Novel coronavirus (COVID-19) outbreak: A review of the current literature. Eurasian Journal of Medicine and Oncology. 2020;**4**:1-7. DOI: 10.14744/ejmo.2020.12220

[5] Rothan HA, Byrareddy SN. The epidemiology and pathogenesis of coronavirus disease (COVID-19) outbreak. Journal of Autoimmunity. DOI: 10.1016/j.jaut.2020.102433

[6] Phelan AL, Katz R, Gostin LO. The novel coronavirus originating in Wuhan, China. Challenges for global health governance. Journal of the American Medical Association. DOI: 10.1001/jama.2020.1097

[7] Woolf SH, Chapman DA, Lee JH. COVID-19 as the leading cause of death in the United States. Journal of the American Medical Association. 2021;**325**:123-124. DOI: 10.1001/jama.2020.24865

[8] Marazuela M, Giustina A, Puig-Domingo M. Endocrine and metabolic aspects of the COVID-19 pandemic. Reviews in Endocrine and Metabolic Disorders. 2020;**21**:495-507. DOI: 10.1007/s11154-020-09569-2

[9] Puig-Domingo M, Marazuela M, Giustina A. COVID-19 and endocrine diseases. A statement from the European Society of Endocrinology. Endocrine. 2020;**68**:2-5. DOI: 10.1007/s12020-020-02294-5

[10] Pal R, Banerjee M. COVID-19 and the endocrine system: Exploring the unexplored. Journal of Endocrinological Investigation. 2020;**43**:1027-1031. DOI: 10.1007/s40618-020-01276-8

[11] dos Santos LR, Filho RB, Alves TAFdA, Jardine MB, Durate ML. Covid-19 and endocrinology-intersections: A review of current knowledge on physiopathological associations. Endocrinology & Metabolism International Journal. 2020;**8**:90-95. DOI: 10.15406/emij.2020.08.00286

[12] Lundholm MD, Poku C, Emanuele N, Emanuele MA, Lopez N. SARS-CoV-2 (COVID-19) and the endocrine system. Journal of the Endocrine Society. 2020;**4**:1-13. DOI: 10.1210/jendso/bvaa144

[13] Arlt W, Baldeweg SE, Pearce SHS, Simpson HL. Endocrinology in the time of COVID-19: Management of adrenal insufficiency. 2020;**183**:G25-G32. DOI: 10.1530/EJE-20-0361

[14] Kothandaraman N, Rengaraj A, Xue B, et al. COVID-19 endocrinopathy with hindsight from SARS. American Journal of Physiology Endocrinology and Metabolism. 2021;**320**:E139-E150. DOI: 10.1152/ajpendo.00480.2020

[15] Alzahrani AS, Mukhtar N, Aljomaiah A, et al. The impact of COVID-19 viral infection on the hypothalamic–pituitary–adrenal axis. Endocrine Practice. 2021;**27**:83-89. DOI: 10.1016/j.eprac.2020.10.014

[16] Fleseriu M, Buchfelder M, Cetas JS, et al. Pituitary society guidance:

Pituitary disease management and patient care recommendations during the COVID-19 pandemic - An international prospective. Pituitary. 2020;**23**:327-337. DOI: 10.1007/s11102-020-01059-7

[17] Wang W, Su X, Ding Y, et al. Thyroid function abnormalities in COVID-19 patients. Frontiers in Endocrinology. 2021;**11**:623792. DOI: 10.3389/fendo.2020.623792

[18] Dworakowska D, Grossman AB. Thyroid disease in the time of COVID-19. Endocrine. 2020;**68**:471-474. DOI: 10.1007/s12020-020-02364-8

[19] Shaha AR. Thyroid surgery during COVID-19 pandemic: Principles and philosophies. Head & Neck. 2020;**42**:1322-1324. DOI: 10.1002/hed.26198

[20] Aojula N, Ready A, Gittoes N, Hassan-Smith Z. Management of parathyroid disease during the COVID-19 pandemic. Journal of Clinical Medicine. 2021;**10**:920. DOI: 10.3390/jcm10050920

[21] Narici M, De Vito G, Franchi M, et al. Impact of sedentarism due to the COVID-19 home confinement on neuromuscular, cardiovascular and metabolic health. Physiological and pathophysiological implications and recommendations for physical and nutritional countermeasures. European Journal of Sport Science. DOI: 10.1080/17461391.2020.1761076

[22] Martinez-Ferran M, de la Guía-Galipienso F, Sanchis-Gomar F, Pareja-Galeano H. Metabolic impacts of confinement during the COVID-19 pandemic due to modified diet and physical activity habits. Nutrients. 2020;**12**:1549. DOI: 10.3390/nu12061549

[23] Wake DJ, Gibb FW, Kar P, et al. Endocrinology in the time of COVID-19: Remodelling diabetes services and emerging innovation. 2020;**183**:G67-G77. DOI: 10.1530/EJE-20-0377

[24] Guo W, Li M, Dong Y, et al. Diabetes is a risk factor for the progression and prognosis of COVID-19. Diabetes Metabolism Research and Reviews. 2020;**36**:e3319. DOI: 10.1002/dmrr.3319

[25] Muniyappa R, Gubbi S. COVID-19 pandemic, coronaviruses, and diabetes mellitus. American Journal of Physiology Endocrinology and Metabolism. 2020;**318**:E736-E741. DOI: 10.1152/ajpendo.00124.2020

[26] Yang M, Chen S, Huang B, et al. Pathological findings in the testes of COVID-19 patients: Clinical implications. European Urology Focus. 2020;**6**:1124-1129. DOI: 10.1016/j.euf.2020.05.009

[27] Li H, Xiao X, Zhang J, et al. Impaired spermatogenesis in COVID-19 patients. EClinicalMedicine. 2020;**28**:100604. DOI: 10.1016/j.eclinm.2020.100604

[28] Achua JK, Chu KY, Ibrahim E, et al. Histopathology and ultrastructural findings of fatal COVID-19 infections on testis. The World Journal of Men's Health. 2021;**39**:65-74. DOI: 10.5534/wjmh.200170

[29] Jing Y, Run-Qian L, Hao-Ran C, et al. Potential influence of COVID-19/ACE2 on the female reproductive system. Molecular Human Reproduction. 2020;**26**:367-373. DOI: 10.1093/molehr/gaaa030

[30] Raghavan D, Tan AR, Story ES, et al. Management changes for patients with endocrine-related cancers in the COVID-19 pandemic. Endocrine-Related Cancer. 2020;**27**:R357-R374. DOI: 10.1530/ERC-20-0229

[31] Popkin BM, Du S, Green WD, et al. Individuals with obesity and COVID-19: A global perspective on the

epidemiology and biological relationships. Obesity Reviews. 2020;**21**:e13128. DOI: 10.1111/obr.13128

[32] Clemmensen C, Peterson MB, Sørensen TIA. Will the COVID-19 pandemic worsen the obesity epidemic? Nature Reviews. Endocrinology. 2020;**16**:469-470. DOI: 10.1038/s41574-020-0387-z

[33] Rychter AM, Zawada A, Ratajczak AE, Dobrowolska A, Krela-Kaźmierczak I. Should patients with obesity be more afraid of COVID-19? Obesity Reviews. 2020;**21**:e13083. DOI: 10.1111/obr.13083

[34] Alberca RW, Oliveira LdM, Branco ACCC, Pereira NZ, Sato MN. Obesity as a risk factor for COVID-19: An overview. Critical Reviews in Food Science and Nutrition. DOI: 10.1080/10408398.2020.1775546

[35] Gao F, Zheng KI, Wang XB, et al. Obesity is a risk factor for greater COVID-19 severity. Diabetes Care. 2020;**43**:e72-e74. DOI: 10.2337/dc20-0682

[36] Kwok S, Adam S, Ho JH, et al. Obesity: A critical risk factor in the COVID-19 pandemic. Clinical Obesity. 2020;**10**:e12403. DOI: 10.1111/cob.12403

[37] Greenway FL, Look M, Golden A, et al. COVID-19 and the urgent need for new therapies for obesity. Population Health Management. DOI: 10.1089/pop.2020.0307

[38] Sorokin AV, Karathanasis SK, Yang ZH, Freeman L, Kotani K, Remaley AT. COVID-19-associated dyslipidemia: Implications for mechanism of impaired resolution and novel therapeutic approaches. The FASEB Journal. 2020;**34**:9843-9853. DOI: 10.1096/fj.202001451

[39] Atmosudigdo IS, Lim MA, Radi B, et al. Dyslipidemia increases the risk of severe COVID-19: A systematic review, meta-analysis, and meta-regression. Clinical Medicine Insights: Endocrinology and Diabetes. 2021;**14**:1-7. DOI: 10.1177/1179551421990675

[40] Clemente-Suárez VJ, Dalamitros AA, Beltran-Velasco AI, Mielgo-Ayuso J, Tornero-Aguilera JF. Social and psychophysiological consequences of the COVID-19 pandemic: An extensive literature review. Frontiers in Psychology. 2020;**11**:580225. DOI: 10.3389/fpsyg.2020.580225

[41] Coelho-Ravagnani CdF, Corgosinho FC, Sanches FLFZ, Prado CMM, Laviano A, Mota JF. Dietary recommendations during the COVID-19 pandemic. Nutrition Reviews. 2020;**79**:382-393. DOI: 10.1093/nutrit/nuaa067

[42] Muscogiuri G, Barrea L, Savastano S, Colao A. Nutritional recommendations for CoVID-19 quarantine. European Journal of Clinical Nutrition. 2020;**74**:850-851. DOI: 10.1038/s41430-020-0635-2

[43] Galanakis CM. The food systems in the era of the coronavirus (COVID-19) pandemic crisis. Foods. 2020;**9**:523. DOI: 10.3390/foods9040523

[44] Gasmi A, Chirumbolo S, Peana M, et al. The role of diet and supplementation of natural products in COVID-19 prevention. Biological Trace Element Research. DOI: 10.1007/s12011-021-02623-3

[45] Lippi G, South AM, Henry BM. Electrolyte imbalances in patients with severe coronavirus disease 2019 (COVID-19). Annals of Clinical Biochemistry. 2020;**57**:262-265. DOI: 10.1177/0004563220922255

[46] Taheri M, Bahrami A, Habibi P, Nouri F. A review on the serum electrolytes and trace elements role in

the pathophysiology of COVID-19. Biological Trace Element Research. DOI: 10.1007/s12011-020-02377-4

[47] Dehghani-Samani A, Kamali M, Hoseinzadeh-Chahkandak F. The role of vitamins on the prevention and/or treatment of COVID-19 infection; A systematic review. Modern Care Journal. 2020;**17**:e104740. DOI: 10.5812/modernc.104740

[48] Jovic TH, Ali SR, Ibrahim N, et al. Could vitamins help in the fight against COVID-19? Nutrients. 2020;**12**:2550. DOI: 10.3390/nu12092550

[49] Belete TM. Review on up-to-date status of candidate vaccines for COVID-19 disease. Infection and Drug Resistance. 2021;**14**:151-161. DOI: 10.2147/IDR.S288877

[50] Xing K, Tu XY, Liu M, et al. Efficacy and safety of COVID-19 vaccines: A systematic review. Chinese Journal of Contemporary Pediatrics. 2021;**23**:221-228. DOI: 10.7499/j.issn.1008-8830.2101133

[51] Doroftei B, Ciobica A, Ilie OD, Maftei R, Ilea C. Mini-review discussing the reliability and efficiency of COVID-19 vaccines. Diagnostics. 2021;**11**:579. DOI: 10.3390/diagnostics11040579

[52] Li Y, Tenchov R, Smoot J, Liu C, Watkins S, Zhou Q. A comprehensive review of the global efforts on COVID-19 vaccine development. ACS Central Science. 2021;**7**:512-533. DOI: 10.1021/acscentsci.1c00120

[53] Kumar A, Dowling WE, Román RG, et al. Status report on COVID-19 vaccines development. Current Infectious Disease Reports. 2021;**23**:9. DOI: 10.1007/s11908-021-00752-3

[54] Gao QY, Chen YX, Fang JY. 2019 novel coronavirus infection and gastrointestinal tract. Journal of Digestive Diseases. DOI: 10.1111/1751-2980.12851

[55] Mousavizadeh L, Ghasemi S. Genotype and phenotype of COVID-19: Their role in pathogenesis. Journal of Microbiology, Immunology and Infection. 2021;**54**:159-163. DOI: 10.1016/j.jmii.2020.03.022

[56] Ammar A, Brach M, Trabelsi K, et al. Effects of COVID-19 home confinement on eating behaviour and physical activity: Results of the ECLB-COVID19 international online survey. Nutrients. 2020;**12**:1583. DOI: 10.3390/nu12061583

[57] Garre-Olmo J, Turró-Garriga O, Martí-Lluch R, et al. Changes in lifestyle resulting from confinement due to COVID-19 and depressive symptomatology: A cross-sectional a population-based study. Comprehensive Psychiatry. 2021;**104**:152214. DOI: 10.1016/j.comppsych.2020.152214

[58] León-Zarceño E, Moreno-Tenas A, Boix Vilella S, García-Naveira A, Serrano-Rosa MA. Habits and psychological factors associated with changes in physical activity due to COVID-19 confinement. Frontiers in Psychology. 2021;**12**:620745. DOI: 10.3389/fpsyg.2021.620745

[59] Gadde KM, Martin CK, Berthoud HR, Heymsfield SB. Obesity. Pathophysiology and management. Journal of the American College of Cardiology. 2018;**71**:69-84. DOI: 10.1016/j.jacc.2017.11.011

[60] Saxon DR, Iwamoto SJ, Mettenbrink CJ, et al. Antiobesity medication use in 2.2 million adults across eight large health care organizations: 2009-2015. Obesity. 2019;**27**:1975-1981. DOI: 10.1002/oby.22581

[61] Heshmati HM. Anti-obesity medical devices. In: Himmerich H, editor.

Weight Management. London: IntechOpen; 2020. p. 239-253. DOI: 10.5772/intechopen.91697

[62] Radvinsky D, Iskandar M, Ferzli G. Bariatric surgery today: The good, the bad, and the ugly. Annals of Laparoscopic and Endoscopic Surgery. 2017;**2**:52. DOI: 10.21037/ales.2017.02.26

[63] Ammar A, Chtourou H, Boukhris O, et al. COVID-19 home confinement negatively impacts social participation and life satisfaction: A worldwide multicenter study. International Journal of Environmental Research and Public Health. 2020;**17**:6237. DOI: 10.3390/ijerph17176237

[64] Bradbury-Jones C, Isham L. The pandemic paradox: The consequences of COVID-19 on domestic violence. Journal of Clinical Nursing. 2020;**29**: 2047-2049. DOI: 10.1111/jocn.15296

[65] Zhang Z, Arshad A, Zhang C, Hussain S, Li W. Unprecedented temporary reduction in global air pollution associated with COVID-19 forced confinement: A continental and city scale analysis. Remote Sensing. 2020;**12**:2420. DOI: 10.3390/rs12152420

[66] Venter ZS, Aunan K, Chowdhury S, Lelieveld J. COVID-19 lockdowns cause global air pollution declines. Proceedings of the National Academy of Sciences. 2020;**117**:18984-18990. DOI: 10.1073/pnas.2006853117

[67] Barua S, Nath SD. The impact of COVID-19 on air pollution: Evidence from global data. Journal of Cleaner Production. 2021;**298**:126755. DOI: 10.1016/j.jclepro.2021.126755

[68] Delang L, Neyts J. Medical treatment options for COVID-19. European Heart Journal: Acute Cardiovascular Care. 2020;**9**:209-214. DOI: 10.1177/2048872620922790

Section 3

Miscellaneous

Chapter 6

Estrogen as a Contributing Factor to the Development of Lipedema

Sara Al-Ghadban, Mary L. Teeler and Bruce A. Bunnell

Abstract

Lipedema is an underdiagnosed painful adipose tissue disorder that occurs almost exclusively in women, with onset manifesting at puberty or at times of hormonal change. Unlike many fat disorders, diet and exercise have little to no impact on the prevention or progression of this disease. Estrogens control the distribution of body fat and food intake, regulate leptin expression, increase insulin sensitivity, and reduce inflammation through signaling pathways mediated by its receptors, estrogen receptor alpha (ERα) and ERβ. This review will focus on understanding the role of estrogen in the pathogenesis of the disease and envisage potential hormonal therapy for lipedema patients.

Keywords: lipedema, adipose tissue, estrogen, adipogenesis, inflammation

1. Introduction

Lipedema is a chronic underrecognized adipose tissue (AT) disorder distinguished by the symmetrical accumulation of painful fat in the lower body, predominantly in the thighs. The clinical presentation of lipedema resembles that of obesity, lymphedema, and other AT disorders, so it is often misdiagnosed and mistreated [1–4]. Lipedema is diagnosed by a thorough physical examination in conjunction with the patient's family and medical histories. Healthcare providers identify lipedema through the following criteria: bilateral and symmetrical distribution of subcutaneous fat predominantly in the legs that excludes the hands or feet, minimal pitting edema and a negative Stemmer's sign which can indicate edema followed by a set of detailed criteria that characterize regionalization of fat accumulation and pain, time of change in fat distribution, and diet resistance to discern the type and stage of the patient.

There are five different types of lipedema, which are based upon the regions of prominent fat deposition. Type 1: the fat builds up in the buttocks and hip; Type 2: the fat spreads from the buttocks to the knees with fat folds around the inside of the knee; Type 3: the fat extends to the hips and ankles, the feet are not affected; Type 4: the fat is increased in the upper arms sparing the wrist and Type 5: the fat accumulates in the lower legs only [2, 5, 6]. Patients may present with more than one type depending on the progression of the disorder. Additionally, patients present at three different stages, depending on the severity of fat accumulation and the onset of other symptoms [2, 5–7]. Stage 1: the skin is smooth with small fat lobules; Stage 2: the skin has indentations with pearl-sized fat nodules and Stage 3: the skin has large extrusions with overhanging fat causing tissue deformities. Lymphedema may also develop collaterally at any stage of the disorder but does not alone qualify a case of lipedema [2]. Unlike many AT disorders, lipedema is largely irresponsive to lifestyle interventions such as diet and exercise, but liposuction and decongestive therapy are effective treatment options [1]. While neither are curative, liposuction is widely accepted as the better treatment option for its ability to provide long-term improvement to appearances, functionality, mobility and bruising while reducing edema, spontaneous pain, sensitivity to pressure. Combined decongestive therapy (CDT) such as pre- or post-operative lymphatic drainage or use of compression garments in recovery weeks may be conducted in support of the procedure [2, 4].

Lipedema predominantly affects females and often manifests during time of hormone fluctuations, during puberty, childbirth, or menopause [7, 8], indicating that estrogen and estrogen signaling play a role in the pathogenesis of lipedema via direct impacts on adipocytes and immune cells, and/or secondary effects on the brain control centers [9, 10]. However, the exact mechanism(s) of action remain unclear [11, 12]. Although lipedema is a common disease (11% of women worldwide), no data are yet available to demonstrate the prevalence of lipedema in pre- and post-menopausal or pregnant women. In addition, cases of lipedema in males are very rare; however, men who develop lipedema tend to have high levels of estrogen but low testosterone levels [2, 5, 6]. Understanding the mechanisms of the life-long transitions of estrogen levels and interactions with AT will define the pathogenesis of lipedema more thoroughly while identifying novel diagnostic and treatment options.

This review will describe the potential role of estrogen in the development of lipedema. The effect(s) of estrogens on the immune system will be described, the association of estrogen signaling on tissue adipogenesis and inflammation will be explored and the application of estrogen as a potential therapy in preventing the progression of this disease will be discussed.

2. Estrogens and estrogen receptors in lipedema

Estrogens are hormones that regulate adipose tissue metabolism by controlling food intake, energy expenditure and body distribution. Estrogens have widespread effects on several organs around the body and therefore play a role in a variety of physiological functions and disorders. Estrogens can act on receptors in both the cytoplasm and the plasma membrane to mediate protein expression involving cell proliferation and metabolism [12]. Estrogens are present in three forms: estrone (E1), estradiol (E2), and estriol (E3). Estradiol is the most extensively studied, as it plays key roles in reproductive phase functioning and a large variety of chronic disorders. There are three receptors that have distinct presences and functions around the body. Alterations in estrogen activity or the absence of estrogen receptors (ER) results in the accumulation of subcutaneous adipose tissue (SAT), a phenomenon observed in lipedema patients [5, 9, 13, 14]. Szél et al. hypothesized that alteration in ERs is involved in the regulation of appetite and weight gain which might explain why lipedema patients accumulate fat and have difficulty losing it with diet and exercise [10]. Furthermore, Yi et al. showed that estrogen regulates the expression of leptin, a hormone that controls hunger and body weight, in adipocytes via ERs [15] supporting the hypothesis that lipedema is a hormonal disease.

Estrogen exerts its function through the estrogen receptor alpha (ERα) and beta (ERβ). Both ERα and ERβ receptors appear in significantly high concentrations in SAT of premenopausal women, as signaling from estrogens mediates adipose deposition throughout the body [9, 16]. However, ERα expression is reduced in the SAT of clinically obese females and postmenopausal women treated with estradiol compared to their normal-weight counterparts [14, 17, 18]. Interestingly, Erβ, which serves an antagonistic role on ERα-mediated gene expression, is highly expressed in postmenopausal women in comparison to premenopausal women [19]. Such findings raise the question of whether a correlation of the concentrations of estrogen receptors in adipose tissue could elucidate a similar relationship between estrogen receptor concentrations in lipedema AT. Additionally, a study conducted by Gavin et al. discovered described that the concentration of ERα is decreased and ERβ concentration is increased in the lower extremities of overweight patients, associating the variable concentrations to sexual dimorphisms in regionalized fat deposition for individuals [20]. As discussed earlier, fat accumulates in the lower extremities of lipedema patients, implying a potential role of ER in its pathogenesis. Furthermore, Dieudonné and colleagues evaluated the expression of ERs in preadipocytes and adipocytes in a cohort of lean subjects and determined that males and females statistically share similar levels of both ERα and ERβ within intraabdominal AT (IAT) and SAT [14]. Females have slightly higher concentrations of ERα and ERβ globally than males. However, when induced with estradiol, expression of ERα in the SAT in females increased significantly more than in IAT. In these same conditions, the SAT in females have a significantly increased expression of ERβ while all other levels of ERβ (IAT in females, SAT and IAT in males) remained the same. Cases of increased regionalized lipid accumulation are closely correlated to estrogen deficiency [21–24]. In contrast, in an estrogen-sufficient state, excess fat is stored in the gluteal-femoral region, rather than the abdominal region. One mechanism has been postulated as a factor in this association is the acute administration of estrogens to postmenopausal women which reduced basal lipolysis in SAT, particularly in the femoral region, further supporting a role for estrogens in regional fat deposition in lipedema patients [25].

The third estrogen receptor, G protein-coupled estrogen receptor (GPER) is expressed on the membrane at lower concentrations in adipose tissue but nonetheless, with several important effects. GPER has been widely studied in regulation of body weight, inflammation, insulin sensitivity, and metabolic dysfunction [26–29]. Several studies demonstrated that mice lacking GPER demonstrate an increase in adiposity (mass and adipocyte size) and decrease in energy expenditure compared to their wild type mice [29–31]. Studies have also shown that the lack of GPER or ERα expression in mice show similar characteristic of metabolic syndrome such as inflammation, obesity, glucose intolerance and insulin resistance [26, 31–34]. Although the actions of estrogens on GPER have not yet been fully elucidated, examining the crosstalk between ERs and estrogen will help understand their function in the development of lipedema.

2.1 Estrogen and adipogenesis

Estrogens have been shown to play a role in gender and regional adiposity. Several studies revealed that women have ~10% more early stage preadipocytes in abdominal SAT and ~35% more in femoral SAT [35, 36]. However, only ERα is expressed in preadipocytes, suggesting a role for estrogen in adipogenesis that is not mediated by the antagonistic mechanisms of ERα and ERβ [16]. Lacasa et al. found the mechanisms involved by which estrogen stimulates preadipocyte proliferation, supporting a role of estrogen in adipogenesis [13, 37]. However, Eaton et al. postulated that local adipocyte-produced estrogen may play a role in preventing preadipocyte differentiation based on data from two studies where treatment of preadipocytes with estrogen, both in vitro and in vivo, inhibited adipogenesis and lipogenic gene expression [13, 38]. The distribution of preadipocytes and adipocytes along with the expression of estrogen receptors on differentiated adipocytes could play a role in the pathogenesis of lipedema, as regionalized and sexually distinct adipocyte hypertrophy is one of the central defining characteristics of the disorder.

Activation of ERα, ERβ, and GPER on adipocytes elicit an intranuclear response, causing up or down-regulation in the expression and activity of proteins such as leptin and lipoprotein lipase (LPL), which are involved in lipid regulation in the body [39, 40]. Through this regulation of protein expression, estrogen partially mediates weight control and lipogenesis-lipolysis mechanisms. Moreover, several studies have shown that estrogen treatment altered the expression of several genes involved in lipogenesis. A study conducted by Homma et al. revealed a negatively controlled estrogen response element in the LPL gene, indicating that estrogen decreases activity of LPL, a protein that regulates lipid uptake by adipocytes and leads to lipogenesis, which inhibits adipose deposition [41]. Another study has shown that estrogen stimulates the expression of leptin in human breast tissue [42]; thus, estrogen might play an important in the regulation of adipose tissue. We have shown that leptin gene expression is increased in adipocytes differentiated in vitro from adipose-derived stem cells obtained from obese lipedema patients compared to the same cells from healthy controls [43]; however, the effect of estrogen on the expression of leptin in lipedema has yet to be determined. Additionally, ERβ has been shown to be a negative regulator of peroxisome proliferator-activated receptor γ (PPARγ), a key transcription factor highly expressed in AT and controls the expression of LPL, glucose transporter type 4 (Glut 4) and leptin; thus, a decrease in ERβ expression increases adipogenesis which is detected in lipedema SAT [43]. However, further studies will be needed to study the correlation between the loss of ERs expression and the increase adiposity in AT disorders.

2.2 Estrogen and inflammation

Estrogen exerts regulatory effects on the immune system through ER-dependent and independent pathways [44], which can be both positive and negative depending on a wide array of factors such as the level of estrogen, expression of ERs, cell types and the environment [45]. Lipedema AT is characterized by hypertrophic adipocytes and activated immune cells such as macrophages and mast cells [46–48]; thus, direct, and indirect cellular interaction through auto- and paracrine secretions of inflammatory cytokines via the ER signal transduction pathway have an immense impact on the tissue function [7, 19, 35]. Several studies have shown that a decrease in estrogen levels results in increased expression of pro-inflammatory cytokines, including interleukins (IL)-6, IL1-β and Tumor Necrosis Factor-alpha (TNF-α) as is the case with women undergoing menopause or oophorectomy [49]. On the other hand, in the case of pregnant women or in women taking ectopic estrogens, suppressed immune responses are observed [48]. Hence, as estrogen levels fluctuate in lipedema patients during their lifetime, the inflammatory signals in the tissue may as well. This correlation between estrogen levels and onset of inflammation could provide insight into the pathophysiology of lipedema-associated inflammation.

3. Potential hormonal therapy

Estrogen is widely known as a central regulator of fat metabolism and regional deposition. In premenopausal women, estrogen is synthesized in the ovaries during menstruation [19]; however, it is depleted as they age. In adipose tissue, androgens are aromatized into estrogens to restore hormonal levels and prevent the progression of hormonal-related diseases [17, 19, 50]. One study found increased aromatase activity in a group of obese individuals, supporting a correlation between this shift of hormone production and metabolic disease [51]. However, estrogen deficiency or depletion, such as in the case of ovariectomy, polycystic ovary syndrome (PCOS), or the lack of a functional aromatase gene, causes weight gain which is associated with comorbidity, cardiovascular disease, and other diseases; thus, hormone replacement therapy (HRT) was shown to be an effective treatment [52–57]. In the context of AT, administration of exogenous estradiol to premenopausal women decreases LPL activity in AT of the lower extremities, which are primarily affected in lipedema [58]. However, another study conducted by Lindberg et al. found that the treatment of postmenopausal women with oral ethinyl estradiol (50 μg/day) for three weeks increased adipose tissue LPL activity in femoral adipocytes [59]. Other studies expand on this, finding that estrogen treatment of adipocytes decreased the expression of genes related to adipogenesis and lipogenesis such as PPAR-γ and LPL [19, 38, 58]. Furthermore, administering estrogen resulted in a significant decrease in LPL activity in adipose tissue [52]. Similarly, Pederson et al. discovered that estrogen treatment almost doubled insulin binding affinity in rat adipocytes. Control rats had 11% weight gain in 7 days whereas estrogen treated rats gained only 4% in the same period. Adipocytes were significantly larger in control rats compared to adipocytes from estrogen substituted rats. Interactions of estrogens with androgens to mediate these processes were also discovered, with two studies observing the effects of HRT that further substantiate an association between androgens and weight gain [54, 60]. Davis et al. reported that administering androgens with estrogens in hormone replacement therapy seemed to antagonize or reduce the effects of estrogens on fat deposition and weight loss. Likewise, Gamberini et al. reported administration of antiandrogens with the typical estrogen dosage results in more efficient weight loss. While the effects of androgens in lipedema cases have been underdefined in this literature review, the pathophysiological effect of androgen therapy implies a treatment option for cases of lipedema. Clinical research has also found that women receiving estrogen HRT have relatively increased protection from metabolic syndrome and decreased AT deposition in the intra-abdominal region [13, 61–64]. Additionally, as mentioned above, post-menopausal clinical subjects developed high levels of inflammatory cytokines had associated decreases in such levels following estrogen treatments [13]. All these data confirm that the physiological impact of estrogen is altered as females passes through reproductive benchmarks, and thus estrogen may be a potential treatment of Lipedema patients.

Furthermore, it has been proposed that activation of ERα can induce the browning of white adipocytes, referred to as beiging, through induction of lipolysis mediated by adipose tissue triglyceride lipase [65]. It is known that premenopausal women have more brown adipose tissue (BAT) and are more sensitive to brown adipose tissue activation than men or postmenopausal women. Selective activation of ERα by pyrazole triol (selective ERα agonist) increased markers of beiging in vitro [65]. The results of this study indicated that selective activation of ERα in adipocytes can induce beiging through the induction of adenosine monophosphate-activated protein kinase (AMPK) mediated lipolysis providing free fatty acids as an energy source to activate Uncoupling protein (UCP)-1 [66]. Another study conducted Yepuru et al. demonstrated that activation of ERβ increases mitochondrial function and energy expenditure; thus, ERβ ligands have anti-obesity and antimetabolic disease effects [67] and might be more beneficial than estradiol treatment which unselectively activates both ERs. In vitro and in vivo studies have suggested that selective ERβ ligand reduces the expression of genes associated with white adipose tissue and promote the expression of genes associated with brown adipose tissue. This ligand additionally increases the mitochondrial oxygen consumption without an increase in physical activity [68]. Additional research is needed to gain insight into whether selectively activating of one estrogen receptor over another confers more benefits than activating both unselectively. Given these results on the selective activation of estrogen receptors, there is an increased effort to characterize specific molecular pathways to induce white adipose tissue browning; thus, presenting another potential treatment for lipedema patients.

4. Conclusion

Lipedema is a severe chronic adipose tissue disorder that affects women worldwide. Although the pathophysiology of the disease has not been fully elucidated, several lines of evidence have suggested estrogen dysfunction may be central to the development of lipedema. The loss of estrogen can additionally induce cardiovascular disease and create an insulin resistant dyslipidemia state that can have long term implications on the metabolic profile of a patient. Thus, studying the role played by estrogen in the processes are involved in the pathogenesis, AT inflammation, fibrosis, and angiogenesis, will provide researchers insights into the mechanism involved in the development of the disease and will help direct future study on hormonal therapy as a form of treatment for lipedema. Through these efforts, the correlation revealed between hormones and adipogenesis in AT will lead to evaluate lipedema as a hormonal disease.

Acknowledgements

This work was funded by a grant from the Lipedema Foundation.

Conflict of interest

The authors declare no conflict of interest.

Author details

Sara Al-Ghadban[1,2]*, Mary L. Teeler[2] and Bruce A. Bunnell[1,2]

1 Department of Microbiology, Immunology and Genetics, University of North Texas Health Science Center, Fort Worth, TX, USA

2 Center for Stem Cell Research and Regenerative Medicine, Tulane University School of Medicine, New Orleans, LA, USA

*Address all correspondence to: sara.ghadban@gmail.com

References

[1] Buck, D.W. and K.L. Herbst, Lipedema: A Relatively Common Disease with Extremely Common Misconceptions. Plast Reconstr Surg Glob Open, 2016. 4(9): p. e1043.

[2] Torre, Y.S., et al., Lipedema: friend and foe. Horm Mol Biol Clin Investig, 2018. 33(1).

[3] Vignes, S., [Lipedema: a misdiagnosed entity]. J Mal Vasc, 2012. 37(4): p. 213-218.

[4] Warren Peled, A. and E.A. Kappos, Lipedema: diagnostic and management challenges. Int J Womens Health, 2016. 8: p. 389-395.

[5] Al-Ghadban, S.H., KL; Bunnell BA, Lipedema: A Painful Adipose Tissue Disorder. Adipose Tissue- An Update, ed. S. L. 2019: IntechOpen.

[6] Buso, G., et al., Lipedema: A Call to Action! Obesity (Silver Spring), 2019. 27(10): p. 1567-1576.

[7] Herbst, K.L., Subcutaneous Adipose Tissue Diseases: Dercum Disease, Lipedema, Familial Multiple Lipomatosis, and Madelung Disease, in Endotext, K.R. Feingold, et al., Editors. 2019, MDText.com, Inc.: South Dartmouth (MA).

[8] Perbeck, L. and S. Mellgrim, [Lipedema an often overlooked but treatable disease]. Lakartidningen, 2017. 114.

[9] Cooke, P.S. and A. Naaz, Role of estrogens in adipocyte development and function. Exp Biol Med (Maywood), 2004. 229(11): p. 1127-1135.

[10] Szél, E., et al., Pathophysiological dilemmas of lipedema. Med Hypotheses, 2014. 83(5): p. 599-606.

[11] Brown, L.M. and D.J. Clegg, Central effects of estradiol in the regulation of food intake, body weight, and adiposity. J Steroid Biochem Mol Biol, 2010. 122 (1-3): p. 65-73.

[12] Monteiro, R., D. Teixeira, and C. Calhau, Estrogen signaling in metabolic inflammation. Mediators Inflamm, 2014. 2014: p. 615917.

[13] Eaton, S.A. and J.K. Sethi, Immunometabolic Links between Estrogen, Adipose Tissue and Female Reproductive Metabolism. Biology, 2019. 8(1): p. 8.

[14] Dieudonné, M.N., et al., Evidence for functional estrogen receptors alpha and beta in human adipose cells: regional specificities and regulation by estrogens. Am J Physiol Cell Physiol, 2004. 286(3): p. C655–C661.

[15] Yi, K.W., et al., Role of estrogen receptor-alpha and -beta in regulating leptin expression in 3T3-L1 adipocytes. Obesity (Silver Spring), 2008. 16(11): p. 2393-2399.

[16] Deroo, B.J., Estrogen receptors and human disease. Journal of Clinical Investigation, 2006. 116(3): p. 561-570.

[17] Meyer, M.R., et al., Obesity, Insulin Resistance and Diabetes: Sex Differences and Role of Estrogen Receptors. Acta Physiol, 2011. 203(1): p. 259-269.

[18] Savva, C. and M. Korach-André, Estrogen Receptor beta (ERβ) Regulation of Lipid Homeostasis-Does Sex Matter? Metabolites, 2020. 10(3).

[19] Monteiro, R., D. Teixeira, and C. Calhau, Estrogen Signaling in Metabolic Inflammation. 2014. 2014: p. 1-20.

[20] Gavin, K.M., E.E. Cooper, and R.C. Hickner, Estrogen receptor protein content is different in abdominal than gluteal subcutaneous adipose tissue of overweight-to-obese premenopausal

women. Metabolism, 2013. 62(8): p. 1180-8.

[21] Espeland, M.A., et al., Effect of postmenopausal hormone therapy on body weight and waist and hip girths. Postmenopausal Estrogen-Progestin Interventions Study Investigators. J Clin Endocrinol Metab, 1997. 82(5): p. 1549-1556.

[22] Gambacciani, M., et al., Body weight, body fat distribution, and hormonal replacement therapy in early postmenopausal women. J Clin Endocrinol Metab, 1997. 82(2): p. 414-417.

[23] Jensen, L.B., et al., Hormone replacement therapy dissociates fat mass and bone mass, and tends to reduce weight gain in early postmenopausal women: a randomized controlled 5-year clinical trial of the Danish Osteoporosis Prevention Study. J Bone Miner Res, 2003. 18(2): p. 333-342.

[24] Kohrt, W.M., A.A. Ehsani, and S.J. Birge, HRT preserves increases in bone mineral density and reductions in body fat after a supervised exercise program. J Appl Physiol (1985), 1998. 84(5): p. 1506-12.

[25] Van Pelt, R.E., et al., Acute modulation of adipose tissue lipolysis by intravenous estrogens. Obesity (Silver Spring), 2006. 14(12): p. 2163-2172.

[26] Prossnitz, E.R. and M. Barton, Signaling, physiological functions and clinical relevance of the G protein-coupled estrogen receptor GPER. Prostaglandins Other Lipid Mediat, 2009. 89(3-4): p. 89-97.

[27] Nadal, A., et al., The role of oestrogens in the adaptation of islets to insulin resistance. J Physiol, 2009. 587(Pt 21): p. 5031-5037.

[28] Hugo, E.R., et al., Bisphenol A at environmentally relevant doses inhibits adiponectin release from human adipose tissue explants and adipocytes. Environ Health Perspect, 2008. 116(12): p. 1642-1647.

[29] Haas, E., et al., Regulatory role of G protein-coupled estrogen receptor for vascular function and obesity. Circ Res, 2009. 104(3): p. 288-291.

[30] Davis, K.E., et al., Sexually dimorphic role of G protein-coupled estrogen receptor (GPER) in modulating energy homeostasis. Horm Behav, 2014. 66(1): p. 196-207.

[31] Sharma, G., et al., GPER deficiency in male mice results in insulin resistance, dyslipidemia, and a proinflammatory state. Endocrinology, 2013. 154(11): p. 4136-4145.

[32] Albanito, L., et al., G protein-coupled receptor 30 (GPR30) mediates gene expression changes and growth response to 17beta-estradiol and selective GPR30 ligand G-1 in ovarian cancer cells. Cancer Res, 2007. 67(4): p. 1859-1866.

[33] Vivacqua, A., et al., G protein-coupled receptor 30 expression is up-regulated by EGF and TGF alpha in estrogen receptor alpha-positive cancer cells. Mol Endocrinol, 2009. 23(11): p. 1815-1826.

[34] Ribas, V., et al., Impaired oxidative metabolism and inflammation are associated with insulin resistance in ERalpha-deficient mice. Am J Physiol Endocrinol Metab, 2010. 298(2): p. E304–E319.

[35] Ghaben, A.L. and P.E. Scherer, Adipogenesis and metabolic health. Nature Reviews Molecular Cell Biology, 2019. 20(4): p. 242-258.

[36] Tchoukalova, Y.D., et al., Sex- and Depot-Dependent Differences in Adipogenesis in Normal-Weight Humans. Obesity, 2010. 18(10): p. 1875-1880.

[37] Lacasa, D., et al., Control of Rat Preadipocyte Adipose Conversion by Ovarian Status: Regional Specificity and Possible Involvement of the Mitogen-Activated Protein Kinase-Dependent and c-fos Signaling Pathways*. Endocrinology, 1997. 138(7): p. 2729-2734.

[38] Jeong, S. and M. Yoon, 17β-Estradiol inhibition of PPARγ-induced adipogenesis and adipocyte-specific gene expression. 2011. 32(2): p. 230-238.

[39] Mayes, J.S. and G.H. Watson, Direct effects of sex steroid hormones on adipose tissues and obesity. Obes Rev, 2004. 5(4): p. 197-216.

[40] Mauvais-Jarvis, F., D.J. Clegg, and A.L. Hevener, The role of estrogens in control of energy balance and glucose homeostasis. Endocr Rev, 2013. 34(3): p. 309-338.

[41] Homma, H., et al., Estrogen suppresses transcription of lipoprotein lipase gene. Existence of a unique estrogen response element on the lipoprotein lipase promoter. J Biol Chem, 2000. 275(15): p. 11404-11411.

[42] Morad, V., A. Abrahamsson, and C. Dabrosin, Estradiol affects extracellular leptin:adiponectin ratio in human breast tissue in vivo. J Clin Endocrinol Metab, 2014. 99(9): p. 3460-3467.

[43] Al-Ghadban, S., et al., Increase in Leptin and PPAR-γ Gene Expression in Lipedema Adipocytes Differentiated in vitro from Adipose-Derived Stem Cells. Cells, 2020. 9(2).

[44] Khan, D. and S. Ansar Ahmed, The Immune System Is a Natural Target for Estrogen Action: Opposing Effects of Estrogen in Two Prototypical Autoimmune Diseases. Front Immunol, 2015. 6: p. 635.

[45] Bereshchenko, O., S. Bruscoli, and C. Riccardi, Glucocorticoids, Sex Hormones, and Immunity. Frontiers in Immunology, 2018. 9(1332).

[46] Fain, J.N., et al., Comparison of the release of adipokines by adipose tissue, adipose tissue matrix, and adipocytes from visceral and subcutaneous abdominal adipose tissues of obese humans. Endocrinology, 2004. 145(5): p. 2273-2282.

[47] Blüher, M., Obesity: global epidemiology and pathogenesis. Nat Rev Endocrinol, 2019. 15(5): p. 288-298.

[48] Al-Ghadban, S., et al., Dilated Blood and Lymphatic Microvessels, Angiogenesis, Increased Macrophages, and Adipocyte Hypertrophy in Lipedema Thigh Skin and Fat Tissue. J Obes, 2019. 2019: p. 8747461.

[49] Stubelius, A., et al., Ovarian hormones in innate inflammation. Immunobiology, 2017.

[50] Burger, H.G., The endocrinology of the menopauseProceedings of Xth International Congress on Hormonal Steroids, Quebec, Canada, 17-21 June 1998. The Journal of Steroid Biochemistry and Molecular Biology, 1999. 69(1-6): p. 31-35.

[51] W.H., C., M. C.R., and S. E.R., Effects of aging and obesity on aromatase activity of human adipose cells. J Clin Endocrinol Metab, 1985. 60: p. 174-177.

[52] Pedersen, S.B., et al., Effects of in vivo estrogen treatment on adipose tissue metabolism and nuclear estrogen receptor binding in isolated rat adipocytes. Mol Cell Endocrinol, 1992. 85(1-2): p. 13-19.

[53] Jones, M.E., et al., Aromatase-deficient (ArKO) mice have a phenotype of increased adiposity. Proc Natl Acad Sci U S A, 2000. 97(23): p. 12735-12740.

[54] Gambineri, A., et al., Obesity and the polycystic ovary syndrome. Int J

Obes Relat Metab Disord, 2002. 26(7): p. 883-896.

[55] Misso, M.L., et al., Cellular and molecular characterization of the adipose phenotype of the aromatase-deficient mouse. Endocrinology, 2003. 144(4): p. 1474-1480.

[56] Takeda, K., et al., Progressive development of insulin resistance phenotype in male mice with complete aromatase (CYP19) deficiency. J Endocrinol, 2003. 176(2): p. 237-246.

[57] Maffei, L., et al., A novel compound heterozygous mutation of the aromatase gene in an adult man: reinforced evidence on the relationship between congenital oestrogen deficiency, adiposity and the metabolic syndrome. Clin Endocrinol (Oxf), 2007. 67(2): p. 218-224.

[58] Price, T.M., et al., Estrogen regulation of adipose tissue lipoprotein lipase--possible mechanism of body fat distribution. Am J Obstet Gynecol, 1998. 178(1 Pt 1): p. 101-107.

[59] Lindberg, U.B., et al., Regional adipose tissue metabolism in postmenopausal women after treatment with exogenous sex steroids. Horm Metab Res, 1990. 22(6): p. 345-351.

[60] Davis, S.R., K.Z. Walker, and B.J. Strauss, Effects of estradiol with and without testosterone on body composition and relationships with lipids in postmenopausal women. Menopause, 2000. 7(6): p. 395-401.

[61] Mauvais-Jarvis, F., Estrogen and androgen receptors: regulators of fuel homeostasis and emerging targets for diabetes and obesity. Trends in Endocrinology & Metabolism, 2011. 22(1): p. 24-33.

[62] Alemany, M., Steroid hormones interrelationships in the metabolic syndrome: An introduction to the ponderostat hypothesis. 2012. 11(3): p. 272-289.

[63] Salpeter, S.R., et al., Meta-analysis: effect of hormone-replacement therapy on components of the metabolic syndrome in postmenopausal women. Diabetes, Obesity and Metabolism, 2006. 8(5): p. 538-554.

[64] Haarbo, J., et al., Postmenopausal hormone replacement therapy prevents central distribution of body fat after menopause. Metabolism - Clinical and Experimental, 1991. 40(12): p. 1323-1326.

[65] Santos, R.S., et al., Activation of estrogen receptor alpha induces beiging of adipocytes. Molecular metabolism, 2018. 18: p. 51-59.

[66] Martínez de Morentin, P.B., et al., Estradiol regulates brown adipose tissue thermogenesis via hypothalamic AMPK. Cell Metab, 2014. 20(1): p. 41-53.

[67] Yepuru, M., et al., Estrogen receptor-{beta}-selective ligands alleviate high-fat diet- and ovariectomy-induced obesity in mice. J Biol Chem, 2010. 285(41): p. 31292-31303.

[68] Ponnusamy, S., et al., Pharmacologic activation of estrogen receptor β increases mitochondrial function, energy expenditure, and brown adipose tissue. FASEB journal: official publication of the Federation of American Societies for Experimental Biology, 2017. 31(1): p. 266-281.